Native American Healing

Native American Healing

HOWARD P. BAD HAND

Keats Publishing

Chicago   New York   San Francisco   Lisbon   London   Madrid   Mexico City
Milan   New Delhi   San Juan   Seoul   Singapore   Sydney   Toronto

Library of Congress Cataloging-in-Publication Data

Bad Hand, Howard P.
    Native American healing / Howard P. Bad Hand.
       p. cm.
    ISBN 0-658-00727-0
     1. Teton Indians—Rites and ceremonies. 2. Teton Indians—Religion.
   3. Teton Indians—Medicine. 4. Healing—Great Plains. I. Title.

    E99.T3 B33 2001
    615.8'82'0899752—dc21   2001035777

Keats Publishing

A Division of The **McGraw-Hill** *Companies*

2 3 4 5 6 7 8 9 0   DOC/DOC   0 9 8 7 6 5 4 3 2

ISBN 0-658-00727-0

This book was set in Bembo by Laurie Young
Printed and bound by R. R. Donnelley—Crawfordsville

Cover design by Laurie Young
Cover illustration by Joe Baker

McGraw-Hill books are available at special quantity discounts to use as premiums and sales promotions, or for use in corporate training programs. For more information, please write to the Director of Special Sales, Professional Publishing, McGraw-Hill, Two Penn Plaza, New York, NY 10121-2298. Or contact your local bookstore.

This book is printed on recycled, acid-free paper.

To the memories of Mary Thunder Hawk;
Christine Chasing In Timber; Joe, Ray, Percy,
Winona, and Roy Bad Hand; Robert Little Hawk;
Dr. Robert L. Curry; Father Richard Pates, S.J.;
Father Ted Zuern, S.J.; Burgess Yellow Cloud;
Annie Yellow Cloud; John G. Kemeny
and all of my People who have gone to the Spirit World.
This book is also for all of those who have shared
and are sharing this life with me now.

CONTENTS

ACKNOWLEDGMENTS

I wish to thank the following for their part in the writing of this book:

Wakan Tanka for giving me life and my relations.

My family, especially Terrie, for the years of love, patience, and forgiveness that led me to consider writing this book.

My daughter Erin for her valuable comments on communicating to a non-Lakota audience and her suggestions on language use and idioms in writing.

My many singing blood and adopted brothers and sisters, and my children (Erin, Erika, Jeremy, and Kristina), who have made the power of music manifest so grandly in life.

My brothers Tom Teegarden and Pat Bad Hand, for the many hours of spiritual singing and questing we have done together.

My brother Paul Henry, for the hours of philosophical inquiry into the grain of sand and the universe.

My relatives and friends whose stories and time spent together appear in this book. Thank you, Uncle Leo, for the many hours of spiritual guidance and questioning that helped me to return to our ways.

My dear friends John and Cindy Cunningham, for the transcriptions of my recorded stories, and for their comments and reviews of the written material that were very supportive and encouraging. Thank you, Cindy, for your part in holding my sanity together!

Elizabeth C. Rosenthal, for helping me to survive Boston and Harvard University. Thank you, Betty, for helping to save my sense of self and for your love and nourishment of me. I am and will be forever grateful.

And my students and fellow spiritual seekers whose curiosity about life and the Sage has brought great acceptance and wonder of the mysteries of life to me.

INTRODUCTION

In the fall of 1999, I was sitting in my office seriously contemplating the next steps to take in my life. As I was reaching for the phone to make a call, it rang. The caller introduced himself as an editor looking for someone to write a book on Native American healing. He'd been referred to me by a friend of a friend. I stalled a bit by listing for him the many things I'd have to consider before I could decide whether I could write such a book. He acknowledged all of my concerns, and told me that his company would publish the book if I agreed to write it. We talked on a few more occasions, and I finally agreed to write this book.

I have started writing this book at least four times and have stopped writing four times. Each time I began this book I found myself drifting, writing academically and somewhat dryly about a dynamic aspect of my life that is neither academic nor rigid in practice.

I began to contemplate why I had undertaken this endeavor in the first place. Would this endeavor leave any benefit to humankind at all? In order to complete this book, I had to come to a place of balance within myself. I had to be comfortable sharing that part of my life that others would consider "Native American healing."

Having arrived at that place, I came to realize that I could not write a book on Native American healing. I could, however, write a book on that part of the Lakota tradition in which I hold a role; that role includes healing, among many other activities.

I reviewed my long-standing beliefs, and I took a long look at my people. I looked at their beliefs and fears about sharing traditions, ceremonies, way of life, rituals, and stories. A certain segment of the Lakota people believe that if anything is shared about our people, especially our spiritual beliefs and practices, those things will be lost. We would lose our identity as a people because we would have given it away. Thus, many of my people have taken a position of no sharing with any non-Lakota. This position has gained great popularity, especially during recent years.

Another segment of the Lakota believe that the only way to preserve and maintain our people's integrity, dignity, and identity as a people is to practice our ways, beliefs, traditions, and spiritual activities openly. Whether or not others see, use, or incorporate any of those things into their own lives, this open self-expression is an affirmation of the dignity, integrity, and strength of the well-being of our people.

Much of what I have learned about life has come from individuals who have taught me to have confidence, dignity, integrity, and perseverance in the ways of our people. In fact, most of my relatives and teachers have taught me to have confidence and respect for the ways of all people. Respecting the teaching of those individuals, I present what follows in this book as a way to share what I have learned. Although I do not want to offend the sensibilities of those amongst our people who fear loss of our culture by the kind of sharing that will be presented in this book, I have a strong commitment to individual growth and development based on the search for and expression of truth. I feel that the only way to convey the truths that I have learned is to share the subjective experiences I have had with my teachers. What I have learned about life through my own experience is mine to share. The development of the ritual processes that I use came from suggestions from those teachers, through visions and dreams, and through the need expressed by the demands of the situations and times in which I found myself.

I intend in this book to take the reader through a ritual based on song. In this ritual, I will use the same processes—namely, storytelling and philosophical inquiry—that were shared with me to help me arrive at the truths I have experienced. The reader, through contemplation, will hopefully do the same.

As I proceed through this ritual, I strongly suggest that the reader refrain from any idea that all Lakota rituals are designed and practiced in this way—they are not. I developed the ritual that is presented in this book over a long period of time. I have used it to help me keep a focus on life and its processes, especially those processes I have learned as holding truth and standing the test of time.

The stories that I present come from time spent with my teachers and from my elders and friends who have faced and continue to face life with me. The stories in most instances are created by me to convey truths from those experiences that I have had with my relatives and friends.

The majority of Lakota ritual and ceremony requires appropriate songs. The songs that I present in this ritual were taught to me by Charlie Kills Enemy, Moses Big Crow, John Strike, Percy Bad Hand, Roy Bad Hand, Willie Bad Hand, Robert Stead, John Around Him, and a few others. Each time I learned a song from any one of these individuals, I was told to remember the song. The common theme of these teachers seemed to be, "Combine the old songs with the new, and find a way to teach these songs to the young ones and to anyone else who is interested so that our way will flourish." This book has presented me with the kind of opportunity that these individuals wanted me to find. Because music is the key part of our rituals, time is spent on the nature and meaning of these songs throughout the book.

The healing process that the reader will be walked through is one that I perceive is within the Lakota tradition as well as within all human tradition. Furthermore, I believe it to be the healing process that exists in all of human culture. The format I use to present the actual healing process is a discussion with a spirit friend. The discussion is done in metaphorical language; the reader should connect with the information presented at the level of his or her own moral and spiritual development.

Once the ritual begins, each following chapter begins with a song. While there are no titles for the actual songs presented,

I have taken the most salient line of each song and presented it as a title for the sake of organization and point of reference.

This writing ends with an encouragement: If there is any one desire that I may have for the readers of this book, it is that any individual who reads this will begin to allow himself the Divine Will of the Creator, the supreme will that exists in all of creation. My desire for those who read the following pages is for them to find meaningful and sublime expression in the lives that they are living.

One must muster up the great courage to go live—life is meant to be lived!

—HOWARD P. BAD HAND
TAOS, NEW MEXICO
JANUARY 2001

1

Ritual and Ceremony

Life on the Rosebud Sioux Reservation in South Dakota is challenging and oftentimes extremely difficult. Making ends meet, having enough to eat, making a living, and sheer survival are daily activities that tend to either numb emotional expression or strengthen it. There are many who have the abilities and means to take the challenges and face them admirably. Likewise, there are many who lack the abilities and means and fail at their purpose in life. While personally experiencing both ends of the spectrum at Rosebud in my youth, life at Rosebud gave me great joy, exhilaration, and cause for celebration. It has been a source of continual amazement to me that the Lakota people, despite their restrictive and limiting relationship to the United States, find ways to entertain themselves and fulfill themselves with an ever-present spiritual wealth.

A great majority of the Lakota people have embraced Christianity, its rituals, and its beliefs as the predominant spiritual expressions of their lives. Many are practicing Catholics, Episcopalians, Baptists, Mormons, Methodists, and Evangelists. Some have even started their own churches and religions, including the Body of Christ Church, which my own family from my father's side helped to organize and create, and participated in.

Others have embraced and have practiced the ways of the Native American Church. This religion has drawn from Christian tenets as well as from various indigenous beliefs and practices. Using peyote as a sacrament and the experience of it as a connection to the sacred world, it has a strong membership on the reservation.

2

Judging by all the religious practices in which I have seen our people indulge themselves, we do seem to love ritual and ceremony!

A small minority of the Lakota with others practice a combination of the traditional Sacred Pipe ways with the Christian practice of their family's choosing. My grandmother, Mary Thunder Hawk, and my uncle and aunt, Leo and Christine Chasing In Timber, who helped raise me from childhood, were by my estimation "Friday and Sunday Catholics." During the rest of the time, my grandmother or my uncle and aunt would take me to Lakota rituals and ceremonies when they occurred.

Up until the mid-1960s, much of the Lakota ritual and ceremonial practices were banned by the U.S. government, either by law or by policy. In the mid-60s, several courageous individuals from the Lakota and Dakota tribes in South Dakota began to openly revive the Sacred Pipe rituals, notably the Sun Dance.

More recently, the Native American Freedom of Religion Act has ensured the safe and open practice of Lakota rituals and ceremonies. Until that law was passed by Congress, the rituals that had survived were practiced in secret—most often, at night. The government watchdogs maintaining the bans were often the Jesuits, Episcopalian priests, ministers, and government police who acted on behalf of the local superintendent of the Bureau of Indian Affairs. If any of these groups knew of a planned ceremony, they actively made an effort to stop it from taking place. So, if a ceremony was happening, and you knew you were going to it, you were hit by a sense of adventure and exhilaration coming from a natural rush of adrenaline—I experienced these as the first "highs" of my life.

The Lakota elders of my youth were caught in the transition between the "old ways" and the blossoming twentieth century. With the technological advances of the time, human endeavor brought into the reservation radio, tape recorders, television, amplified sound, and the like. Through these media, other parts of the world were being experienced as never before. New ways of thinking, new sounds, new music, new faces, and new languages were being presented to the old people.

I had the good fortune of having spent a great deal of time with some of the elders learning about the "old ways." Listening to them and their responses to new developments, to their complaints about contemporary times, and the possible effects of both on the Lakota people became a favorite pastime of mine. During those times I spent with the elders, I rarely heard an English word used to describe their experiences and thinking. At the ceremonies and rituals to which I was taken to participate, Lakota

3

was the language of choice. It was spoken with great pride and eloquence.

I spent some time in my youngest years with my father at Red Leaf Community, just south of Norris, South Dakota, on the western border of the Rosebud Reservation. In my memory, I do not have a linear recall of that time. I only have memories of experiences and events that have affected my life. Ceremony and ritual were ever-present from the earliest days of my life. The first ceremony that I recall having attended was held at the home of my paternal grandmother, Annie Yellow Cloud. Many community members of Red Leaf were present. As I was a child at the time, the people attending were not interesting to me in and of themselves; rather my attention was riveted by what I saw them doing. As the people gathered, I saw old men stand up, respectfully address the gathering, and sit down. Many elderly gentlemen and women each seemed to have their say. A few hand drums were brought out, and the whole crowd of people began to sing in unison to the beat of the drums. Not only was the sound of the gathering loud, the songs were moving and beautiful.

After the initial singing ceased, there was quiet. Some men brought out rawhide bundles in which there were very sharply pointed carved bone instruments. These bone carvings were handed to men and women, including my aunts, Winona and Adele. A man started a song, others joined in, and the individuals with the bone instruments went to the center of the circle. They cut the sleeves of their shirts, knelt down, and began to cut into their arms. Taking pieces of flesh off their arms, they wrapped their cut flesh with red cloth.

4

As I watched this, I started to cry. I ran to my Aunt Winona to see what was going on before they could grab me. My cousin Ray, Aunt Winona's son, a little younger than myself, ran with me to her. As we got to her, I could see a look of determination, and what I can now describe as reverence, shining forth from her. She looked at us, smiled, and said everything was okay. What she said to us then took me many years to understand. The words I use to describe what I heard her say are not exactly what she said at the time, but I will share with you as closely as possible what I remember her saying. These are the words I pondered for many years:

> "*Tohanl Wakan Tanka taku nitawa hci ki he yak'u hantan nas* (When you offer to Great Spirit the only thing you truly own), *he nita wocekiye was'ake hci ki he eye* (it is your most powerful prayer). *Wakan Tanka nanihun nan woayupte nic'u kte* (Great Spirit will hear you and answer you)."

5
L♥

Ray and I stood by her until my Uncle Percy came for us to return to a place amongst the crowd. There was much more singing and speaking, but Ray and I and the other cousins went off to play. I never knew how they ended the ceremony. No one ever told me why they had that ceremony, or even what they called it. The little of it that I remember still sticks in my mind. It was and is still a powerful experience in my life.

One spring, I was told that I was to become *Hunka* with a Dawson No Horse from Wakpamni Lake Community on the Pine Ridge Reservation. *Hunka* is the Lakota name for the relationship-making ceremony, one of the seven sacred rituals of the

Sacred Pipe of the Lakota. In the early days after the gift of the Sacred Pipe from the White Buffalo Calf Woman to the Lakota (a story I will tell you shortly), this ritual was given to the Lakota as one of the rites associated directly with the practice of the Pipe ways. I was told by the elders that the ritual was initially used to make certain that no one was without parents or relations; there should always be someone present to take care of a person should their blood relations die, or in some other way become unable to fulfill the functions of the blood relationship. The *Hunka* is considered a most sacred relationship. Those entering such a relationship must vow to hold the relationship with their will in a sacred manner for the duration of their lives. At the time I was told that I would be *Hunka* with Dawson, I did not understand this, but it was explained to me, and I was told that I was to respect and honor the relationship.

After I was prepared for the *Hunka* with Dawson, a *Wacipi* (dance celebration) was organized in Red Leaf. Many of our friends and relatives from the Pine Ridge Reservation were invited and were all present for the celebration. Before the actual dance celebration started, sometime in the late morning, I was dressed in clean clothing, a blanket was wrapped around my shoulders, and I was put on a horse. My father led me on the horse into the center of the gathering of people. As we approached the center, a group of men started a song that had the beat of a parade song. My father slowed the horse and started to walk rhythmically to the beat of the drum. When we stopped, the men finished the song.

An older gentleman with a loud voice known as an *Eyapaha* (an announcer or crier) began to shout, presenting me to the

6

crowd. He told them what we were doing. An even older man stood up with a Sacred Pipe. He spoke a few words and he started to load his pipe. A song was sung as he was doing this, and when he finished, the song was concluded. He went on to say things about the sacredness of the pipe. He explained this *Hunka* ritual that was associated with it. He said we did it a certain way in the past, but now we had to do it this way. He turned to Dawson and offered him the pipe, which Dawson took and lit. Dawson turned to me and took me off the horse. He touched me with the pipe while saying some relational words in Lakota. He blew some smoke onto my head, then he handed the pipe back to the old man. Dawson took the eagle feather that my father had, and he tied it onto my hair. He looked at me intensely and told me that I was now his son. He said, "Call me *Ate* (Father) now from this day on." He turned to the crowd and reaffirmed my name, *Hohe Kte*.

7

The group of singers started to sing an honor song for me, to which Dawson and I danced. We went around in a circle with support from our families dancing behind us. When the song was finished, my family gave Dawson the horse that I was riding along with some other gifts. My family had a giveaway for the gathered crowd, and a feast was given in my honor. By the time the dance celebration started, I was back into my world of singing and dancing. Again, it was exciting and exhilarating!

Till the day that Dawson died, I called him *Ate*. Before his death, he had become a world champion traditional dancer, an influential spiritual leader, and a *Wicasa Wakan* (powerful holy man) amongst the Oglala. He, too, taught me many things during his life about Lakota belief, ceremony, and ritual.

Going to a night ceremony with *Unci* (Grandmother) Mary was always an adventure. If my uncle and aunt could not pick us up by car to go to the ceremony, Grandma would tell me that we would walk. She would gather up some shawls and a blanket or two. Whether the ceremony was a mile or many miles away, we would get on the road walking. Often, someone would see us on the road and give us a ride close to the ceremony. Sometimes, it would take us a few hours to arrive at the site of the ceremony, but when we arrived someone would always greet us. They would sit us down at the table, offer coffee, soup, and bread to us, and catch up on news of family and future activities. They always seemed to talk about those things that potentially affected the people we knew. Meanwhile, singers and other families would begin arriving.

As this was going on, a room would be cleared of all furniture. The participants' blankets and pillows would be placed on the bare floor. Anything metal or reflective would be removed from the room. The windows, if any, in the room would be covered so that no light could enter or leave the room. A blanket to cover the doorway into the room was also prepared to be used when the ceremony started.

As the room was being cleared, a man or woman, usually the helper of the holy man (or medicine man, or spiritual leader), would thoroughly smudge the room, first with sage, and then with cedar. Then some bundles of sage would be brought into the room. One bundle was left by the doorway for participants. One was to take a stem of sage to put on oneself during the ritual. The other bundles were taken apart. The sage was spread out, making a bedding in a circle leaning toward the west side of the room. This I learned later was the beginning of creating the sacred space where the ceremonial leader would do his work. The Lakota call this the *Owanka,* the resting place, or place of appearance (Figure 1.1).

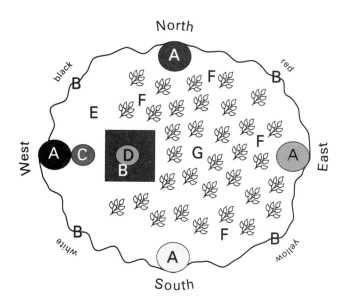

9

A. Cardinal points and corresponding colors.

B. *Canli Wapahta* (tobacco ties with corresponding colored cloths).

C. Sacred objects and feathers.

D. Earth altar on rawhide, newspaper, or cardboard.

E. Sacred food placement.

F. Sage in the *Owanka.*

G. Spiritual leader.

FIGURE 1.1. *OWANKA*
(RESTING PLACE, PLACE OF APPEARANCE)

Outside of the house, men and women would be busy chopping wood. They tended the fire while cooking food to be eaten for the feast at the end of the ceremony. Others would be busy looking for solid, fine dirt to fill up five empty coffee cans. These were used on the *Owanka* as directional markers created for the holy man. In each can of dirt, a stripped chokecherry branch or a dowel would be planted. Usually, two cans were placed toward the westerly direction of the *Owanka,* and one can each in the other three cardinal directions. On each stick or branch, a square yard of cotton cloth with tobacco clumped in one corner was tied. A black cloth was used for the west, a red cloth for the north, a yellow cloth for the east, and a white cloth for the south. Sometimes, a turquoise-green cloth was used in place of the white. The fifth can, placed toward the west, was used for the color cloth of the leader, sacred objects, medicine, and eagle feathers. Just on the inside of the two cans to the west, a piece of cardboard, old newspapers or magazines, or a large leather hide was laid out flat. On this space was placed fine dirt, usually taken from a molehill.

As the people filed into the room, I noticed that the holy man would direct an elderly woman to sit behind him outside of the circle or a young girl to sit in front of him outside of the circle. She would hold the Sacred Pipe throughout the ceremony after it was filled with tobacco. The woman holding the pipe had to be a virgin or a virtuous woman, because she represented White Buffalo Calf Woman in the ritual.

The singers with rawhide hand drums would sit together, usually on the west and north sides of the room. The individual or individuals for whom the ceremony was being conducted were directed to sit on the west side of the room facing the spir-

itual leader. The rest of us would find a comfortable spot any-
where, adjust our blankets and pillows, and sit down preparing for
a long night. At least two persons usually would stay outside, one
apparently watching for unexpected visitors, the other tending
the food and fire.

Most of the night ceremonies that I attended were called
Lowanpi (singing). Once the ceremony began, you were told the
specific kind of ceremony it was that you were participating in.

In my youth, the five predominant categories of ceremony
in the *Lowanpi* were: *Iktomi* (Spider), *Yuwipi* (Bound Up), *Heyoka*
(Clown), *Wanagi* (Ghost or Shadow), and *Wanbli* (Eagle). In practice, there were many similarities in the rituals of each category,
except for the usage of colors of flags, use of the Sacred Pipe,
and the number of tobacco ties used for each ceremony. (Until
I attended Joey Eagle Elk's *Heyoka* ceremony, I was not aware
that the *Heyoka* used the Sacred Pipe. In each *Heyoka* ceremony
I attended before his, the Sacred Pipe was noticeably absent.)

It is important to realize that these categories I mention are
ceremonies that I attended; they are not the only categories of
ritual and ceremony that exist among the Lakota, I am certain.
I have been told of other ceremonies with different names and
purposes. I do not mention them here because I have not been
present at them to know. I have also been told by my grandfathers and grandmothers that many individuals in the early to
middle part of the twentieth century practiced the "old ways" and
healing ways without use of the Sacred Pipe. Many felt that the
Sacred Pipe was too sacred a tool for them to use for mundane
matters. It seems that the use and practice of the rituals and ceremonies of the Sacred Pipe and the further development of the

11

philosophy of the Sacred Pipe have come from the current living generations of the Lakota people. I have wondered often if the ancient people were connected to shamanic traditions that are no longer available to our people today.

What is important is that the Sacred Pipe and the rituals associated with it have become the focal point for some of us. The ways of the Sacred Pipe have become more sacred and a greater responsibility for us, especially for those of us who were raised with some connection to the traditions and the past of our people. The practice and philosophy of the Sacred Pipe have become our way, our belief, and our tradition. I am certain that we do not do what our forefathers did with the *Canunpa,* the Sacred Pipe. All dynamic systems require change. We are in the midst of change and transformation with our traditions, practices, and beliefs. However, the truths I have learned about humanity and life from my people, especially from the old ones, have been solidly consistent and enduring.

I have digressed a bit from my original story, but what I have told you is tied to my experience of the *Lowanpi.* As the holy man put a blanket and sometimes a pillow in the center of the *Owanka* to sit or lie on, a man took a roll of tobacco ties offered by the participants to the holy man. Unrolling them, the man began to lay them on the floor, encircling the *Owanka.*

The *Canli Wapahta* (tobacco ties) are one-inch-square cloth pieces on which tobacco is laid, then wrapped into a pouch, and tied on a string with other like pouches to produce a string of prayer ties. Each pouch of tobacco that is tied to the string is considered a prayer. Based on the requirements established by the holy man, any number of prayer ties, from one to hundreds, can be tied to the string. To keep the ties from tangling with each other, they are rolled into a ball.

The man with the roll of tobacco ties encircling the *Owanka* would always start in the west with black ties, then he would unroll red ties for the north, yellow for the east, and white or green for the south. When he came to the south, he would lay the roll down until the holy man had finished his activities, including filling the *Canunpa*.

The holy man, as he was being encircled, began to unroll *Canli Wapahta* that he had. He would take them, and lay them by the mound of dirt that was laid on the piece of leather or paper. He would turn his attention to the fine dirt that was before him. He would say, "*Ho. Wana Hocokan ki wecagin kte lo!* (Now, I will fix my altar, or center for the voice!)" Everyone in the room would quiet down briefly.

The holy man would first take the sacred food offerings to the Spirits from his helper, and put them next to the dirt mound. These offerings consisted of cut pieces of raw liver, unsugared chokecherry juice, and pounded and shredded meat mixed with fat juices and sugar called *Wasna. Wasna,* also known as pemmican, serves the same purpose as candy.

The holy man would then turn his attention to the fine dirt mound. He would rub his hand on the mound to flatten it, then shape it into a circle. He would take, in most cases, a white eagle feather to smooth out the surface of the circular, flattened earth. He would turn the eagle feather to the pointed side, lean over the circle, and begin to draw symbols or pictures on the fine dirt. The most common symbol I saw, with variations, was a face. Figure 1.2 shows an example.

13

Having finished this drawing, the holy man would take the *Canli Wapahta* (tobacco ties) that he had unrolled, and lay them down, encircling the earth mound. Then, he would say, "*Ho. Letan waceunkiyapi kte lo!* (Now, from here we will pray!)" The holy man's helper would go one more time around the room smudging everyone with sweet grass or cedar. The holy man would ask,

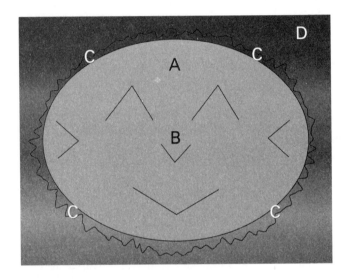

A. Earth mound shaped into circle.

B. Face drawn on the earth.

C. *Canli Wapahta* (tobacco ties).

D. Rawhide, newspaper, or cardboard.

FIGURE 1.2. *HOCOKAN*
(ALTAR, CENTER FOR THE VOICE)

"Iyuha ungluuwinyanpi hwo? (Have we all prepared?)" Everyone would voice their agreement. Men would say *"Hau!"* The women would say *"Haye!"* And there would be lots of laughter.

The holy man would then unroll a bundle that was by his side, which contained his *Canunpa Wakan* (Sacred Pipe), and other sacred objects. He would pull up his pipe bag that contained his tobacco. In some instances, he would take a handful of tobacco, put it on top of a drum, and have his helper pass pinches of tobacco out to everyone in the room. He would say a few words about prayer and the intent of the ceremony we were about to do. He would have everyone do a silent prayer, then have the tobacco picked up again to use to fill the pipe.

In most cases, the spiritual leader would burn rolled leaves of sage by the *Hocokan,* and take a handful of tobacco and smudge it with the smoke of the *Peji Hota* (sage). Then taking one pinch, he would hold it over the burning sage for a moment, point the sage toward the west, say a prayer, and then begin to put it in the *Canunpa.* As he was doing this, the *Canunpa Ojuyapi Olowan* (Pipe-Filling Song) would be sung. He would go through the motions of addressing every direction with the same procedure. He would point to *Wankata* (the heavens), and then point to *Unci Maka* (the earth). When he finished loading the *Canunpa,* he would cap it off with rolled sage. Putting *Tatanka Wigli* (buffalo fat) on the sage to hold it in place on the pipe, he would stand up, holding the *Canunpa.* Offering it upwards, he would sing a song to the Spirit People asking them to acknowledge the sacred activity that we were about to begin. As he finished singing the song, the lamps would be extinguished, and the whole room would go pitch black.

15

The holy man out of the darkness would say a little prayer or a few words to the gathering. Then, he would state that he had a reason why he was doing this ceremonial work, and his rights to do this work. He would begin to recount his *Woihanble* (vision) from which came his direction, skills, or power.

When the holy man finished his story, the helper would strike a match and relight the lamp. Because we did not have electricity in our homes at the time, someone had to be ready to relight the lamp when it was called for. Then, with the lamp now illuminating the room again, the holy man would ask his helper to prepare him for the work that he had to do.

If he was a *Yuwipi Wicasa* (Bound Man), the helper at this point would tie the holy man's hands behind his back. Then, the helper would throw a star blanket over him and wrap him inside the blanket with twine or rope. When this was done, the helper would take the holy man and lay him face down within the *Owanka*. From inside the blanket, the holy man would then ask the light to be turned out. The singing would then be started by the lead singer in the room. This person was usually an older man who had been asked to do this job. Sometimes, the songs would be led by the person who remembered all the songs for this occasion.

If the holy man worked as an *Iktomi Wicasa* (Spider Man), *Wanbli Wicasa* (Eagle Man), or *Wanagi Wicasa* (Ghost or Shadow Man), a different action was taken. Upon the light being turned up, it was time to hand the filled *Canunpa* to the older or young woman who was asked to hold the *Canunpa* for the ceremony. Until much later in my teens, I did not see a *Heyoka* (Clown) use the pipe in a ceremony. But once the *Canunpa* was given to the representative of the *Pte San Win* (White Buffalo Calf Woman), the lights were turned off, and the singing would begin.

As the singing turned into a full chorus of voices, you could hear the holy man sing, shout sacred words to the Spirit World, and intone his own chants invoking the Spirit helpers to come and make an appearance. He would repeatedly state that he needed their help. When finally, as the appropriate songs were sung and each section of ceremony was completed, a change in atmosphere or energy would occur. The holy man would say to us that the Spirit People had now come, and that it was time to state our purpose for being present at the ceremony. Usually, this meant that the people who were sponsoring the ceremony would say their prayers first asking for specific help. Then, each and every person in the room would be asked to say a prayer individually and openly. When this was completed, more songs called *Woayupte Olowan* (Response or Talking Songs) would be sung, then it would be the Spirits' turn to speak to the gathered individuals. It seemed as though every person who said a prayer or asked for something would receive a response.

17

After the responses were given by the Spirit People, usually with some guidance about what to do after the ceremony, the Spirits were returned to the Spirit World. Appropriate songs would be sung to close the ceremony, and the holy man would ask for the lamp to be lit and turned up.

The room became visible again with a few differences. The *Owanka* would be a mess! The smoothed dirt mound would be shapeless and mixed with the tobacco ties. Some of the holy man's items from his *Wounye* (flags) would be missing out of the *Owanka,* but usually in someone's hand. The holy man would appear to be calm, but obviously he had worked very hard at what he had been doing.

The blanket over the doorway would be removed, the door opened, and food would be brought in. Everyone would bring out their dishes. The young men in the gathering would take the food and pass it around. As people ate, there would be words of appreciation spoken, and some of the elders would give a little speech reaffirming the events that had just taken place. Then, as the food was eaten, the sponsoring people would rise and have a *Waihpeya* (giveaway of gifts) to those who had been helpful in the ceremony. Everyone at the end had to say *"Mitakuwe Oyas'in"* before they could leave the ceremony.

18

Grandma and I would catch a ride home. We would arrive home by the time the sun was shining confidently on everything.

I want to share with you what I have learned from these experiences with many different kinds of people in ritual and ceremony. Because I have been participating in these types of ceremonies all my life, I can accept them as one of the enduring aspects of the Lakota culture. And I can also accept them as the helpful processes that my people turn to for many things that affect their lives daily.

Why do we do these rituals and ceremonies? I have spent years wondering about this question. I have arrived at some answers for myself. I will pass these on to you for your contemplation.

The Lakota people face a world that is uncertain, difficult, and challenging. Yet, there is a confidence that prevails that there are ways to meet and resolve these challenges for some benefit. Although it is true that a certain material poverty exists, the people still hold on to a philosophy of sharing and honoring relationships that nourishes and sustains a strong identity and well-being.

Ritual and ceremony provide a way for the people to find peace, harmony, well-being, and wisdom in relating to their environment, as well as helping them make a connection to the Spirit World. At the least, ritual and ceremony allow people to connect with what is real and important. At the practical level, ceremonies give individuals an opportunity to humble themselves and ask for help when it becomes certain that individual effort will not address or resolve the issue or problem at hand. When the request for many hands and minds to be put together for help is successfully met, many things become possible.

A majority of the help requested through ceremony is directly connected to relationship and its resolution. Whether the problems of relationship are personal, intimate, familial, professional, or spiritual, they find their way to the holy man and to the altar. Even before the ceremony begins, the holy man must look at what is presented to assess whether there is harmony, opposition, conflict, or mutuality in the conditions unfolding. When a thorough understanding is achieved, this is shared with the Spirit World so that the direction or guidance given may in turn be thoroughly understood and transmitted to the affected individuals.

Occasionally, an individual may ask for help to heal an injury or cure an illness or disease. The Lakota believe that for every imbalance in health, there exists a guidance or process to balance it. Whether plants and herbs are used, whether the Spirit World gives a spontaneous regeneration of the life forces leading to a healing as well as a cure, or whether guidance or direction is given to use the medical profession to fix or remove

19

something, there is always a potential solution to a situation. This area of work is tricky for the holy man or healer, because great faith is required for positive results from the ceremony. Often when a person asks too late for help from this kind of process, the Spiritual Leader stands the chance of taking on more than can be handled. Though not impossible, it is difficult for a ritual or ceremony to achieve a healing and a cure for a person who is already badly damaged, injured, and decayed by an illness or disease. In these types of situations, the holy man has to put any potential results, success or failure, back into the realm of *Tunkasila* where spontaneous occurrence generates all possibilities. Then whatever is meant to be, will be. Of course, this is always done with a hope for a miracle. And miracles sometimes do happen!

20

I have participated in rituals where the purpose stated for the ceremony was to find lost articles or people, or to take a peek into the future. One of the dangers of simply looking at the future is that one's future might actually be shaped by what is desired from what is glimpsed. It is far better to use what is potential from that view into the future to shape a reality that aligns with truth. Also, what is perceived from the Spirit World is in metaphor. So, without clarity and understanding, a literal view of the future can miss the mark and cause great trouble. It is always good to remember that metaphor contains all potential meaning of the situation to which it is attributed. Many potentials of the same future can be perceived, and they are all possible. The future is conditioned by the past, present, and spontaneous occurrence. It is by looking at the effects of all actions and decisions of the past and present that one can arrive at a true perception of the future being conditioned. In ceremony, this is the information that is always fed back to the people.

When someone has lost something or a person, and is seeking to find this object or person, the seeker is allowed to look into the future to see the potential outcome of his or her search. Many surprises manifest as long as one remembers to look at and accept what is, and also remembers the rules!

There is an abundance of reasons why people would want to participate in ritual and ceremony. You may have realized from these examples that you can do a ritual and ceremony for practically any matter in existence!

I have been the recipient of many opportunities to do ritual and ceremony. I have observed certain patterns that become evident as many rituals are completed. In order to give you a proper look at some of these, it is important for me to share many observations with you about what I perceive as our Lakota people's approach to the practice of our *Woecun* (ways).

First of all, the Lakota use ritual and ceremony as an opportunity to get together with others usually of like mind. This opportunity is treated as an occasion to get help, or in some cases, mutual help. The help most often sought is the help of the Spirit World and the help that can come from that source for a healing. Because many hands and minds are needed to do large ceremonies, many seek the help of each other that can result in great and harmonious accomplishments.

Lakota people believe that the process of ritual and ceremony is the best place to unite all of the religious forces necessary for people to unite appropriately. However, to unite appropriately requires a human leader to serve as the focal point of gatherings that are to be used as a means to get in touch with the sacred. It appears that the Lakota place a great responsibility upon such a leader. This leader must be centered, that is, collected within himself. Through this leader, a collective agreement is reached whereby the mundane and the Spirit World are brought together. Nothing great can happen until this agreement is reached. When this agreement is reached a crystallization of religious forces occurs, the bond between the people is strengthened, and correct action is set into motion.

A final reason the Lakota use ritual and ceremony is the opportunity to share the abundance of a few with the many. Many ceremonies are requested simply to say "*Wopila* (Thank you)," or to show appreciation for good fortune and abundance received. The ceremony provides an opportunity for those gifted with abundance to share the wealth and enhance and further the virtue of kindness.

The focal point of our ceremony, the ceremony of this book, is to share the power of prayer and wisdom to nourish your heart and mind. We do this through song.

The setting of our ceremony is a large room with all windows and openings covered to keep out physical light. The *Owanka* that I sit at does not have a floor covering of sage as done in the past. However, the *Wounye* (flags) of the four cardinal directions are present. The *Owanka* is encircled with 405 tobacco ties and the *Hocokan* (altar) is encircled by 85 tobacco ties of my color, turquoise-green, and a mixture of the four cardinal colors with a number of orange ties. My sacred objects along with my pipe lie on a space above the *Hocokan*. Without going into detail about the symbols on the *Hocokan,* I will show you what is on the dirt face of the altar. (See Figure 1.3.)

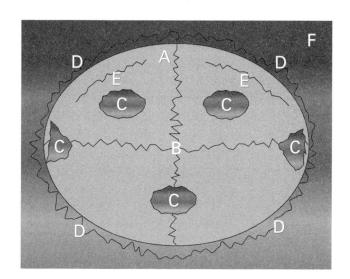

A. Earth mound shaped into circle.

B. Cruciform made with tobacco.

C. Face made with tobacco.

D. Tobacco ties of different colors.

E. Lightning streaks made of tobacco.

F. Rawhide, newspaper, or cardboard.

FIGURE 1.3. *HOCOKAN*
(ALTAR, CENTER FOR THE VOICE)

My *Wounye* (flag), which is used at all of my ceremonies, is a turquoise-green cloth strip, six inches wide by three feet long. It has sixteen tobacco ties of the same color cloth tied to one of its corners. It hangs on a dowel stick just inside the west's black flag.

I sit on a plushy pillow in the center of the *Owanka* (just in case I fall asleep)!

I prepare my pipe. I start the *Canunpa Opagin Olowan* (Pipe-Filling Song), and load the pipe with a mix of tobacco and herbs. I finish loading the pipe. The room is darkened. I tell you my vision from which this *Hocokan* comes. I share my prayer for this ceremony with you.

24

> *Tunkasila, unsimalayo* (Grandfather, have pity upon me). *Wocekiye wan unkagapi ke le* (This prayer that we are making), *Mitakuwe ki lenan ninpi wacin yelo* (I want my relatives here to live). *Ca, heun waceunkiya pelo* (So, we are praying together for this reason). *Wowahwala, Wotakuye, Wicozani, nanhan, Wicouncage unyuha pi kte lo* (We will have Tranquillity, Harmony, Well-being, and Proper Development). *Unninpi ki le unnic'u pelo* (We give to you our lives).
>
> *O unkiya po* (Help us).
>
> *Mitakuwe ob iyuskinyan wani kte lo* (I, with all my relations, will joyfully live)!

The light in the room is turned back on. I hand my pipe to the woman chosen to hold the pipe, giving her instructions to be aware of any phenomena that may happen to her during the ceremony while she is holding the pipe. She must share these phenomena with me if anything occurs during the ceremony. I turn my attention back to the *Hocokan* as the helper for this ceremony ties the tobacco ties together, closing the circle of the *Owanka*. We are ready to begin singing. The room is darkened again.

We will now continue with our ceremony. . . .

2

The Music and Its Role

The music that the Lakota thrive on in ceremony is vocal music supported by percussion. The percussion is provided predominantly by rawhide drums and rattles. Occasionally melody support is provided by eagle bone whistles. A ceremony can sometimes be conducted entirely by the vocal music without the percussion.

As I was growing older, and I began to understand the music of our people, I also began to notice that many of our spiritual leaders, shamans, medicine people, holy people, and visionaries came from the ranks of natural musicians. I once asked my Grandma Mary why this was so. She told me, "*Olowan nayah'un ki lena Tunkasila tawa ye!* (These songs that you hear belong to Grandfather!) *Tuwa Tunkasila kici was'agya wocekiya un woglaka cin hantan nas* (If someone through prayer wants to speak strongly with Grandfather), *kilowan hantan nas* (if he sings to 'Him'), *woayupte wan okoyake ye* (an answer is tied to it)! *Ca Tunkasila nanih'un yacin hantan nas* (If you want Grandfather to hear you), *Ta olowan ki unspe ic'iciya ye* (teach yourself His songs)! *Tuwa lowan hantan nas* (If someone sings), *Tunkasila nakicih'un ye* (Grandfather hears for him)!"

I heard many elders compare, share, and argue about songs. The common theme seemed to be that song is the language used by *Tunkasila* and the Spirit World to communicate to our world. A person who could catch a song, compose a song, or learn a song had easier access to the sacred. One might suppose that a natural musician had a head start to the *Wakan!*

28

Today, much of the sacred music that I listened to and heard in ceremony as a child is not sung, not learned, nor in vogue. Young healers and spiritual leaders still rely on music for the practice of their rituals, but Sun Dance songs predominate over the older, "appropriate" songs. I find myself often puzzled by this phenomenon. Is there a fault here of the old people not leaving their knowledge behind for these younger practitioners? Or is it that the younger spiritual leaders are simply recapturing their sense of being Lakota through the sacred songs of the world that they grew up in?

I do not perceive this as an issue of right or wrong. I do believe that my generation and the generations following mine are doing the best that is possible given the challenges and pressures of our time. I have given this development of current sacred music much thought. People of my generation, including myself, would love to affect the learning of the young people in the most positive ways affordable. Many of us have been taught to honor and respect the old. Personally, I have not been taught to become attached to the old, but rather to learn from the old their ideals that operate as today's realities. I have been told to face today with the best that is within me. If enough people from my generation can do that, they will find that our ideals will operate as tomorrow's realities that our younger generations will have to contend with. The young ones today will leave their ideals for the following generations to experience and contend with. The least resistant path by which this happens is created by music.

The music that touches you deeply, to your core, connects the past, present, and future in the current moment in such a manner that when you allow your being to merge with it, a true reality is created and experienced by you. Without enhancement by drugs or external means, your physical being is released of tension and disharmony. You may respond with movement, dance, enthusiasm, inspiration, or creativity, but you will respond! This is what I believe the elders meant when they said that music is the language of *Tunkasila* or of creation.

It appears that everything that we human beings do is somehow intrinsically tied to music in some form. At the very least, we hang on to our past with music and live in the present moment with music. Do we create our future with music? I believe that we can and actually do! In moments of harmony and inspiration motivated by our response to music, we delve into our ideals and begin to put energy into making them real. They begin to be more real as we hang on to them. Our future finds itself in the present, and we have shaped the future!

The Bad Hand family is a family of singers. We are aware of at least five generations of singers in this family. That I was born into this family, I consider one of *Tunkasila's* great gifts to me. I started singing with my family publicly quite early in my childhood. I gained my experience in music and singing with my family primarily at *Wacipis* (dance celebrations) now known as powwows. I grew up learning the popular music of our people, composed many popular songs, and shared and performed music with many relatives and friends around the world. I did not think of our family as doing much within the sacred realm. Until twenty years ago, I thought our family's music was performed only in the secular arena of our people. I was pleasantly surprised by the truth!

In the late 1970s, I found out that my Uncle Percy Bad Hand was returning to the *Hocokan* (altar) after many years of absence from the practice. I knew him to be a firm believer in the Bible. He loved to study it, and talk about his understanding of the "Great Book." He helped to organize and participated in the development and creation of the Body of Christ Church, which had many followers on the Rosebud and Pine Ridge Reservations. So, when I learned of the path he was returning to, I was surprised.

Until the late 1970s, I did not know of the wealth of sacred music within our own family, nor did I know of Uncle Percy's previous position as a holy man. I only learned of this when I participated in an *Inipi* (purification lodge) with him. In that lodge, he and my brothers sang songs that I was totally unfamiliar with. The experience became a "Sing now, learn later!" proposition! I thought I was well versed in sacred song tradition of our people until that day of our purification. The valuable lesson I learned, which sticks with me today, is the power of music in ritual and ceremony.

30

In that particular *Inipi,* even songs that I knew were sung with different words than the ones I was familiar with. I learned from that particular ceremony that when you have a living, dynamic language, you use words in your music that relate to the moment you are performing the music! The song melodies that I had known were the same, but they were sung with note variations and definitely with differences in style. Of course, some songs were sung that were totally different to me. And songs that I did know were not sung in the order that I had learned them. I realized that it was not a liturgy that I had learned, but only an expression of the reality of that present moment. That momentary confusion had me laughing at myself!

From that *Inipi,* I realized that every holy man who has a ceremony will draw from the generic songs known by a large number of people, but as the ceremony gets to be more specific, more songs are recalled, created, and sung for that particular moment. The holy man may even have his own particular songs for certain spirits, events, and situations. I asked my Uncle Percy why he thought this was so. Recalling his own past, he told me that his father, grandfathers, and grandmothers had always told him that the *Woihanble* (vision or dream) that a holy man gets from the Spirit World is particular to that person. It has directions, boundaries, rules, and conditions that belong only to the person with that vision. No one else can gain power and authority from that vision. So all the activity directed by that vision may have its own songs and goals that the person receiving it must follow in order to maintain the proper connection to the Spirit World. He said that it could not be given away or owned, though connection to it could be lost by the recipient's own actions and decisions. He said, "Your vision is yours to help the world with. Only you can get stronger in it. The only reason why you share the vision in ceremony is that people must know how your way and influence in spiritual matters started. They must also know why you must stay on your course. Your vision will show them that truth. When the Spirits give you songs, you must sing those songs to help the people. Don't worry if they learn them or not —you have to know those songs! Someone should always know these songs. They help us live!"

I left that *Inipi* thinking of the sacredness of song. The more I thought about the songs, the more I was also drawn by the word usage in those songs. What is word in a song? What is going on here?

One day after I received a cassette tape of sacred songs from another uncle, Charlie Kills Enemy, I started to write down the words that I was hearing in the songs so that I could remember them. I had received copies of tapes before from Moses Big Crow, so I had had the experience of listening to tapes from which I could learn the words. In this particular moment of listening to Uncle Charlie's vocal style and rendition of the songs, rather than just listening to them to memorize by rote, I was moved to pay more attention to the meaning of the words. As I penciled each word, I began to have sudden realizations as to why the particular words were used. Whether the words were from the past, or just created for the ceremony about to take place, a pattern was beginning to emerge in my mind showing me the real value of the word usage. I was being directed in how to see the world, spirit, and material, and I was also being directed in how to think of the reality of the present moment.

There are certain words used in sacred songs repeatedly. They are almost always metaphorical, and they carry great meaning.

Wakan Tanka is most often translated into English as "Great Spirit." If one looks at the root words in Lakota that make this name, one begins to see a bit more than just Great Spirit. *"Wa"* is the word that describes an action to be taken into something. *"Kan"* is the word that describes a vein through which blood flows, or the nerves that carry life's energy throughout the body. Of course, a vein is a pathway by which life fluid is carried through the human, plant, or animal body. *"Wakan"* is then translated into English as "sacred." *"Tanka"* means large, grand, or great. The two words put together in the holy people's understanding would translate into "action into the pathway of life in its grandest." The implication of this is enormous—we are creation's grandest vehicle for the expression of life. We are connected to all of life in this way. By the word *"kan,"* this truth is expressed in ourselves. It is saying that each of us expresses the creator through our lives. The creator is not "out there," we express the creator in ourself.

Tunkasila is translated into English as "Grandfather." In Lakota, this word describes many things: the patriarch of a family; the oldest and most revered male individuals in a *Tiospaye* (large family or community); someone in high authority, such as the president of the United States; and the Grandfather of Creation. The word *"tun"* means birth. The word *"ka"* is derived from *"kan"* meaning old or ancient. *"Si"* describes somewhat of an "in-law" relationship. *"La"* describes a very familial affectionate relationship. Together, the root words would describe the most loving relationship to ancient birth, meaning a direct

33

connection to the ancestors or those who have come and gone before us.

Unci Maka is popularly translated as "Grandmother Earth." *"Un"* means to be or living as being. *"Ci"* comes from *"cin"* meaning want, desire to, and will to. *"Maka"* means earth or dirt. The words together convey the earth willing to live, which implies "living earth as mother to all."

Unsimala can be understood as "love me" or "pity me." Again the root word *"un"* means living, or to make use of. *"Si"* means to have a relationship that is binding in some way. *"Ma"* refers to me or myself. *"La"* describes close affection. The meaning then conveyed by the whole word is akin to saying, "Live in the closest relationship with me."

Wayanka as a word joined with a command or assertion conveys the meaning of "look upon, perceive, or make an appearance."

Mitakuwe (ye) is translated as "my relations," usually of blood. Coupled with *"ye"* the word means relations that are made by action or by request.

Oyas'in carries the meaning of "inclusive of all." Together with the word *"mitakuwe,"* the phrase *"mitakuwe oyas'in"* has a meaning that conveys "my blood relations inclusive of all."

Owanka is understood today roughly as a "resting place." The word came originally from *"owayanka"* which originally meant "a place to see, or a place of making an appearance."

Ocokan means "within the center." *"O"* means in or within. *"Co"* is a word meaning keen, smooth. *"Kan"* means "ancient, old." The whole word then conveys a meaning of "smoothness from the ancient." For the Lakota, this means "centering in smoothness."

Hocokan seems to be more of a modern word made up of two words together. *"Ho"* means the voice. *"Cokan"* means the center. The meaning can then be expressed as either the "center voice," or as the "center for the voice." Today, the translation identifies the "altar."

As I pondered on the words most commonly used in our music, a cosmology that was shaped far before my time began to emerge clearly. But I was beginning to understand that these words were used simply to describe a reality about how things really are and how things really work. The music that these words were attached to only helped to make one aware of these simple truths.

In bringing the potential wisdom contained in the words to life, the music in ceremony was doing its part! When sacred, meaningful words are attached to songs that are performed in a harmonious and unobstructed relationship, the past, present, and future, and all who are in that reality with you, are brought together. In the material as well as the spiritual world, this is what I experienced while growing up. It is still my present experience. I have confidence that this will continue until the Spirit World beckons me to make my journey there!

In the Lakota traditional world of today, the secular and the spiritual activities undertaken by the people draw on what is perceived as "old" or traditional, all the while creating new practices to meet the needs of our times. From what the elders have told me, this is the way it has always been.

While in my youth, I encountered many people, young and old, who were very critical of their contemporaries for not doing things "right." There was a sense of conflict always present with these people, and at the least, they were constantly in

35

opposition to any of the activities that the communities on our reservation were embarking on.

In a few experiences that I had with some of them, especially those who did not agree with things that I was doing or believed in, I drew up the courage to say to them that if I did not know how to do things right, they should show me what is right! What I experienced from them was very enlightening. Their responses ran the extremes from discounting me totally, to sitting me down and showing me "how to do things right." A few of them even said to me, "This is how you should be a Lakota." As they proceeded to share their views and beliefs with me, what was curious to me was that those who took the time to try to convince me all had dissimilar views and beliefs. The experiences made me wonder who was right. I began to shape my views of the world from the wealth of wisdom I was being offered even if I did not agree with all of it.

One of creation's wonderful gifts to me is music. I started to sing publicly with my cousin Ray at the age of three; he was also nearly three at the time. He and I were always at the sides of our uncles and fathers, especially when they were singing in public gatherings. So Ray and I naturally started singing. Playing outside of our homes, we would find a large coffee can. Turning it upside down, we would fashion some drumsticks out of sticks we had found. Pounding the can to keep rhythm, we would sing our favorite songs that we had heard from our fathers and uncles. Our fathers and uncles must have heard us a few times, because they started to invite us to sit with them at the drum when they were singing.

We went to the Annual Pine Ridge Oglala Celebration shortly after Ray and I turned three. There, during the dance, the announcer, John Fire, asked the people to clear the dance ground so that they could hear the future of Lakota music. He embellished a great story about song and dance. Then he told the people that two great singers would perform for them.

A family named Black Elk came forward and asked John to ask the two singers to honor a family member of theirs who had been wounded during the Second World War. So, John asked the people to dance for this veteran when these singers sang his honor song. I should have been paying attention!

The man, Black Elk, who was to be honored with song was known by his Lakota traditional name, *O O Sakowin* (Wounded Seven Times). When a warrior or veteran is honored with song, he is named in the song with a little metaphorical story about his service. So, when singers are asked to sing for someone, they must pay attention to find out who they are to sing for. Obviously, neither Ray nor I was paying attention, because after John Fire recounted a little history of *O O Sakowin,* he said that these two gifted singers would now be brought to the center of the dance ground to sing this honor song. He called Ray and me out to the center of the dance ground. I was surprised, and I'm sure Ray was too. But I knew that he wanted to sing, because I certainly did.

Our fathers grabbed a hand drum (it was a big drum to Ray and me) and took us out to the center. They grabbed a few cut logs that we could use as chairs. Ray and I sat down facing each other, and they put the drum between us. My father handed me a drumstick and Ray got one, too. Uncle Percy started to hum a tune to give us an idea of what to sing. We beat him to the punch—we already knew what we were going to sing.

We started to sing. The people stood up and began to dance. The song we were singing started out okay. Everything

37

was fine until we had to sing *O O Sakowin*. We got to the *O* part and repeated *O O O O O,* . . . until John leaned over and said the name correctly to us. We stopped, and started the whole song again. This process took us four tries before we sang the name correctly. When we did get it right, we sang the song numerous times in triumph. The people seemed to be having a great time. When the song was completed, the people, especially *O O Sakowin's* family, had a big giveaway to us. I remember lots of sweets and soda pop, and I thought if this is what singing gets you, I was going to do lots more of it!

In the mid 1950s, Uncle Percy took Ray, me, my brothers, and some cousins to some *Wacipis* (dance celebrations) under the name Red Leaf Takoja. The name stuck, and the name of the group has become known worldwide.

Ray and I, with our relations, sang together until his passing in the early 1970s. Our singing together allowed us to learn about many traditions and traditional songs. What turned out to be even more exciting was when we learned that we could "catch" songs. We found that we could make songs happen as well as compose them. And as the new songs were sung, people would develop activities around them and do things they had not done before. In effect, bringing new songs into the circle was helping people create new traditions. From this, I began to understand that a singer's role in the Lakota way is not only to hold songs, but to create them. This directly helps the people develop new traditions around them.

Having grown up a singer, my experience with critical and obstructive people took a strange twist in my teens. I had made a song that was liked by my family and friends who sang with us.

So for a summer of *Wacipis,* we sang that song on numerous occasions. The song caught on, and it became a popular hit in the Intertribal Dance celebrations and competitions. The song had words that described the joy and love of dancing. We were constantly asked to sing the song wherever we went to sing.

On one of those occasions I asked a person to show me the correct way of doing something, and the individual began to emphatically defend his view of what correctness meant. In his intensity to show me the correct way of doing things in the Lakota way, he said, "Let me give you an example of what I mean about people not doing things right. Last winter, I made a song that everyone sings now. They sing the words of that song this way (he sang to me the words I had fit into my song). It should be sung this way!" He proceeded to sing my own song back to me in the "correct" way! I listened to him finish the song. "See what I mean?" he asked.

I looked at him. After some silence on my part, I said to him, "What you've been telling me would make a whole lot of sense if I felt that you were telling me the truth. What you just sang to me is my song. Can you tell me here, now, that you made that song, and not me?" Because I was not sure if I was angry, confused, or puzzled, I was sincere in trying to get him to look at what he had just shared with me. The look on his face made me wonder if we were about to do battle with each other.

The man softened his look, began to walk away, and said over his shoulder, "I was just kidding you!"

The majority of my learning experiences about the music of our people was far more encouraging and supportive than just being told how to do it "right." As I was getting into my

39

teens, my family of singers began to spread out to other parts of South Dakota and Nebraska, so the opportunities to sing as a family began to dwindle. However, as the small community dance celebrations were the main means of expressing our traditions, there was much gathering and tribal support for the numerous *Tiospaye* of our people in their celebrations. So, there were many occasions for me to sing. I would often be taken by family to these celebrations throughout the northern plains to go dance and sing.

In the small communities of Rosebud, the celebrations were supported by longtime singers and dancers. If I arrived at a celebration without my family singing group, some older singers such as Sievert Young Bear, Dave Clairmont, Leo Clairmont, Frances Menard, John Strike, and Ben Black Bear among others would ask me to sit down with them at the drum to sing. Sievert especially enjoyed my toying with melodies of new songs. He would "buy" new songs from me to encourage my growing repertoire. So, much more encouragement from these singers, aside from my own family's encouragement, helped fan the creative side of my singing life. They would always pique my interest in traditional songs as well. As a child, I grew up learning many songs from older singers that I had heard, and with *Tunkasila's* gift of memory to me, I remembered a lot of songs. These older singers considered me an equal as a singer despite the difference in our ages. They took pleasure in making me feel good about *Tunkasila's* gifts to me. One particular truth that they felt I should remember and would always emphasize to me was that our people and our ways would die if our music died. I took this to heart—our music is the source of our pleasure and life!

Uncle Charlie Kills Enemy thoroughly encouraged the singing tradition that I was raised in. He would send my brother Tom or me tapes of sacred music. He would have a commentary about the music on the tape. He once said about a particular cassette tape that I still have in my possession, "These songs should be learned and understood in the proper way. Boys and girls should learn how to sing the sacred songs. If we lose the sacred songs as a part of our Indian culture, the Indian culture will die! We should help each other sing these songs, so that all of our prayers will be effective." He was always of the opinion that the songs carried our sacred language, so the Spirits would respond to these with the sacred language.

Every singer who has ever taught me a song that is sacred gave it with the understanding that this is true communication with *Tunkasila* and the Spirit World. All sacred songs should be sung with that intention and understanding. This is true of all the sacred songs, whether they are "old" or new compositions.

Until very recently, the Lakota separated their sacred music from their secular music. The sacred language used in ceremonial settings was not taken into the secular settings, and the same was true in reverse. I remember my father and uncles sang a song in an early 1970s New Year's celebration in St. Francis, South Dakota. It was so powerful that people who were dancing went into a frenzy over it for nearly an hour. After the song was over, two of my uncles remembered that two sacred songs they knew sounded so much like the new song they had sung that they vowed to never sing that song again in public. I have sung that song in a few different dances since then, but they never did sing that song again.

41

For the young people of today, especially in interaction with other tribes around the country, sacred language has crept into dance celebration songs as artistic interpretations and compositions. Even songs composed for the powwows have found their way into sweat lodges, Sun Dances, and other sacred arenas without taboo.

In my personal life, this kind of composition has inspired me to compose or catch songs from the universe that contain sacred language but have found homes in the dance celebrations. Two examples of this exist for all to hear in public.

The first song, which the Dine (Navajo) elders from the Big Mountain area were gifted with song from the Spirit People through me, has these words in both Lakota and Navajo: *Tunkasila yapi* (president of the United States, and Grandfather of Creation). *Wamanyanka yo* (Look upon me). *Le miye ca, tehiya nawajin yelo* (It is I standing here having a difficult time). *Unci Maka nawecinjin nan wowahwala wan, kuwa waun welo* (I defend Grandmother Earth, and I live seeking peace). This song has been sung in both sacred and secular celebrations.

The other song containing sacred language that is now a big part of the secular dance celebration world was requested of me by the Denver March Powwow, Inc., of Denver, Colorado. I sincerely believe that the Spirit People gave me this song to give to the people of Denver March Powwow. The song is sung at every grand entry of the three-day song and dance event. It contains these words: *He Ska Oyate ki!* (White Mountain People!). *Oskate ki le luha pi ki, Cangleska ca nin un welo* (This celebration that you have is a living hoop). *Sitomniya, Tunkasila nan Unci Maka ko, oniciya pi nan iyuskinya waci a u welo* (From the universe, even Grandfather Creator and Grandmother Earth help you, and all come joyfully to dance). The song's original title was *A Living Hoop,* but it is popularly known as the Denver March Powwow Song.

My meeting Arlie Neskahi and his family inspired me to compose a few secular dance songs with sacred language to emphasize beauty and harmony in the relationship between all beings. Ingenious word usage by Arlie in many of his songs and my being moved by his melodies and words opened up a whole new world of song for me. Where taboo existed before about uniting the sacred with the secular, at least for a few, this taboo no longer exists.

The older sacred songs are still available to be learned by the younger spiritual leaders. The area of great creative song making among the Lakota has come within the last decade, especially in the Sun Dance circle. These songs sing praises to *Unci Maka* (Grandmother Earth) and *Tunkasila,* to a new life returning, and they give thanks for all of the good things in life. It appears that the younger generation of Lakota and other tribes are feeding off this great creativity. So, in the current ceremonial circles and *Inipi* lodges, much more Sun Dance music is sung. The old people have said to us that we should make use of the old songs in the most productive means possible, otherwise their usefulness is gone and they die out. Enough older songs are sung along with the new ones to make the tradition of song have a vibrant life. I also feel that books like this one will help us connect appropriately with the past.

For the ceremony that you are now entering in this book, we are singing the old and new songs together. According to the singers who have taught me much of the music being shared with you now, the songs that you will experience are in the following categories: *Canunpa Ojuyapi Olowan* (Pipe-Filling Song), *Canunpa Opagin Olowan* (Pipe-Offering Song), *Tatioye Topa Olowan* (Four Directions Song), *Wakan Tanka Taolowan* (Great Spirit Song), *Lel Etunwan Yo* (Personal Sacred Song), *Wicakicopi Olowan* (Spirit Calling Songs), *Tiuma Hiyupi Olowan* (Spirit Entrance Songs), *Wakan Ki Wacipi Olowan* (Spirit Dancing Songs), *Wakan Ki Woglakapi Olowan* (Spirit Talking Songs), *Wakan Woayupte Olowan* (Spirit Responding Song), *Wakan Kinanpe Olowan* (Spirit Departure Song), *Wakan Wicak'upi Olowan* (Offering Song), *Woawanyanke Olowan* (Protection Song), and *Wakan Iglustanpi Olowan* (Ceremony Completion Song). There are other categories of songs, but we will only use the songs given above for our ceremony.

Let us sing!

44
♪♥

3

Friend, Do It This Way

Kola, lecel ecun wo.	Friend, do it this way.
Kola, lecel ecun wo.	Friend, do it this way.
Kola, lecel ecun wo.	Friend, do it this way.
Lecanu ki,	If you do it this way,
Ni Tunkasila,	Your Grandfather,
Wani yank u kte lo.	Will come to see you.
Owakan wanji,	In a resting place,
Yuha ilotake ce,	(when) You sit down with it,
Mi ksu ya wacekiya yo.	Remember me as you pray.
Ecanu ki,	If you do that,
Ni Tunkasila,	Your Grandfather,
Wani yank u kte lo.	Will come to see you.
Kola, lecel ecun wo.	Friend, do it this way.
Kola, lecel ecun wo.	Friend, do it this way.

Kola, lecel ecun wo.	Friend, do it this way.
Lecanu ki,	If you do it this way,
Ni Tunkasila,	Your Grandfather,
Wani yank u kte lo.	Will come to see you.
Hocokan wanji,	A center place for your voice,
Yuha ilotake ce,	(when) You sit down with it,
Mi ksuya hoye kiya yo.	Remember me as you send your voice.
Ecanu ki,	If you do that,
Ni Tunkasila,	Your Grandfather,
Wani yank u kte lo.	Will come to see you.
Kola, lecel ecun wo.	Friend, do it this way.
Kola, lecel ecun wo.	Friend, do it this way.
Kola, lecel ecun wo.	Friend, do it this way.
Lecanu ki,	If you do it this way.
Ni Tunkasila,	Your Grandfather,
Wani yank u kte lo.	Will come to see you.
Canunpa wanji,	A (sacred) Pipe,
Yuha ilotake ce,	(when) You sit down with it,
Mi ksuya opagin yo.	Remember me as you offer the smoke.
Lecanu ki,	If you do this,
Taku yacin ki,	Whatever you will (or want),
Ecetu kte lo.	Will be so.

This song is sung as the holy man begins his prayer in preparation to load his *Canunpa.* The song continues until he is finished. He addresses the directions as he puts *Kiniknik,* or tobacco mix, into the pipe bowl, a pinch at a time for each direction and for the animal or force of nature attributed to each. In his prayer, he invokes *Wakan Tanka*. He invokes *Tunkasila*.

The song itself, "Friend, do it this way. If you do it this way, your Grandfather will come to see you," carries a greater meaning than just the words of Grandfather coming to see you. Again, the word *Tunkasila* means the closest relationship that exists between you and all that preceded you, the past. This ideal "Grandfather coming to see you" points out that all that was before, is now, and the potential of the future is what you are about to experience. So, the song says, "In this place of rest, when you sit down, remember me as you pray." This refers to the Spirit talking to the holy man. Through the song, the Spirit is saying, "Remember me and all that was before you, what is now, and what can be in the future. Remember this as you pray. Again, if you do this, your Grandfather will come to see you."

Most of the singing for this song usually only addresses a *Canunpa* (the Sacred Pipe), or the *Owanka* (the resting place). But in the Lakota tradition, sometimes the singer adds other words to signify the connection to the present moment—what we are doing in the here and now. And so, in our song here, we address the center place. We address the altar, the place where your voice is spoken to the Spirit World. Of course, the Spirit in the song is saying, "In this place of your voice, when you sit down there, with this pipe, remember me as you send your voice. Again Grandfather will come to see you. Friend, if you do it this way, your Grandfather will come to see you." And then, literally, the song says, "When you sit down with this Sacred Pipe, remember me as you offer this smoke. If you do this, whatever

47

you will, or want, will be so." This song, purely on the idea of the literal, shows that the Spirit is talking to the holy man, looking in on the connection that he is about to make to the Spirit World. The Spirit World is saying, "If you do it this way, connect to the past, the present, and the future, then all that is potential will become visible, will become manifest." This is what is presented in the song.

"Do it this way" is a metaphor for a way of being, a way of acting, a way of behavior. What I learned from the old people about the gift of the Sacred Pipe was that the gift came at a high point in the development of our warrior tradition. It was given to us at a time when we began to treat war as a game. The chase for power and glory predominated over spiritual considerations. A few of the elders that I grew up listening to thought that the gift from the Spirit of the *Canunpa* was a true spiritual gift to the Lakota people, which caused them to look at a more feasible and appropriate reality that began to connect the people back to the Great Spirit.

When there is a highly idealized expression of the warrior tradition, the warrior tradition treats war as a game. It becomes a focal point for the gain of glory. It becomes a point of recognition of oneself within that warrior society. But with the introduction of the Sacred Pipe, the Lakota were given a different way of seeing the world, and a different way of acting. They were shown a way of behavior, that, if one looks at the metaphor and what it includes, began to challenge the people to return to a life in balance and in harmony with the Spirit World and the material world, where this game of war was being played out.

I listened to the older people talk about this sacred gift. They talked about the gift of the Sacred Pipe, the *Canunpa*. They

48

talked about *Pte San Win*, the White Buffalo Calf Woman, coming to the Lakota people with the Sacred Pipe. The first appearance she made was to two warriors who had been away from the village for days, walking, looking for game, and hunting in order to take food back to the people in the village. As they were walking on the prairie, they saw what appeared to be a very bright colored object approaching them from the distance. At first, it looked like a buffalo. As they approached it, they began to realize that it was a young, beautiful maiden dressed in a very white, clean buckskin dress. An encounter between the three became inevitable. Mystified, the two warriors looked at each other. The first warrior began to think of all the things that could happen there in the wide open plains with this young, beautiful maiden they saw approaching. He told his friend, "We should take her." This meant sexually overpowering her to satisfy his physical needs. The other warrior, the younger of the two, hesitated. He thought this was too strange that a young woman would be walking alone, without fear, in the middle of the plains and coming toward them. So, he tried to restrain his friend from even thinking of taking the young woman. He said to his partner, "This is a *Wakan* situation, something beyond the ordinary. It is not wise to go after this young maiden in the way that you are thinking of doing!"

The first warrior did not listen to the younger warrior. The story goes that the foolish brave went after the White Buffalo Calf Woman. He approached her and encountered her. The old people say that dust and smoke began to surround the two of them. Winds came up. The younger warrior stood back in amazement and fear. He simply watched what was going on.

49

When the smoke and dust cleared, the White Buffalo Calf Woman was still standing. The young warrior who had tried to restrain his friend looked to where his friend had once stood. What he saw was that his warrior partner had been reduced to rubble. Snakes were eating at his flesh, and his body was disintegrating before his very eyes.

The young warrior decided to humble himself in front of this *Wakan* woman. Young warriors were taught that such an encounter with the *Wakan* can be very dangerous. One can lose one's life if the *Wakan* is not treated appropriately. So, the young warrior humbly asked for forgiveness for himself and for his friend. By this time, the first warrior had been reduced to the earth. The younger warrior truly begged for his life.

White Buffalo Calf Woman looked at the young warrior. She told him to return to his people with a message for them to prepare a large lodge where they all could be gathered. She would come and offer to the people a gift from the Spirit. The gift would be brought, she said, to bring peace, to bring harmony, to bring well-being (in the sense of justice), and to bring wisdom to the people.

The young warrior took this message to heart. He rushed back to his village and told the elders what the White Buffalo Calf Woman had said. The elders realized this could be nothing other than a true sacred event. They prepared a large lodge for the White Buffalo Calf Woman, who was to come with the gift in a few days.

The story, with its strong message, was one that I was told and asked to contemplate frequently. What is this story really telling the Lakota people? The Lakota language carries meaning sometimes far beyond the literal, so I did not contemplate this in terms of the literalness of the story, or the mythology of the story, but of its true meaning. I was encouraged by the elder people to think of the story in this fashion.

Initially, the warriors were on a journey with a good cause. They were to go out and take the life of an animal to bring back to the people, so the people could be fed, could be nourished. They were to do this, so that the people would live.

So, with this cause, these two warriors set out. The elders have told me that it is important to remember that these two were warriors. I was also told to be mindful of the warrior's sense of the sacred; the acceptance of the sacred is a very small part of the thinking of the warriors in their activity.

"In encountering the sacred," an elder named Sam Bear told me, "look at these two. One stepped back from what he perceived as truly a situation beyond the normal. A young woman without fear, with true confidence, is walking across the plains, first appearing to be a buffalo. That attracted the warriors' attention. When the warriors realized what they saw was indeed a young beautiful maiden, they drew on their greatest weakness, that weakness being passion. One warrior was moved to act on his passion. The other had to step back in reason, and look at the situation in its unfolding. The warrior with the passion was so intent in his aggression to own the young woman that his own passions and his own weaknesses caused him to disintegrate.

"The other warrior rationally began to look at this, began to humble himself, and began to put himself below the young maiden." And Grandpa Sam said, "If you look at this story in this way, you will see that the first message ever taught by the

51

White Buffalo Calf Woman, in encountering these two warriors, is for you to be very careful of your intentions. When you learn to humble yourself, to create harmony with the situation, you begin to regain life. And in regaining life, the sacred entrusts you with the message of what is to come—the gift of Spirit that gives you life."

So, I have always looked at this song, "Friend, Do It This Way," as encouragement to act in an appropriate and beneficial way, not only for yourself, but for all people. The message of a better life, a promise of a better life, becomes evident when you return your life to humility and appropriate action to accept the sacred, the connection to the Spirit World where *Tunkasila* resides.

In this world, *Unci Maka,* from which all living things are born and nourished, bears with all that life in its unfolding presents to her. Grandpa Sam Bear, along with other elders along the way, encouraged me to begin to look at this as a story that contained more than just the literal progression to receiving the gift of the Sacred Pipe.

Many look at this story simply as a literal event in which two young warriors encountered the White Buffalo Calf Woman. From this came the gift of the Sacred Pipe, but the gift of the pipe occurred much later than the actual encounter. The older people who used to recount this story to me always said, "Look at what we were being shown and directed to do." They did not talk of process. They did not talk of how this was to be done. They just said, "Look at this. Think about this. What was given to us with this *Canunpa?*"

As I grew older, I realized that these sacred songs had a greater meaning and message, not only in the performance, but in the history and the directions for living that they carried. I began to look at stories that were being shared with me in a much different way. I also realized quite early in life that the warrior way, in and of itself, was not the way to spiritual understanding, acceptance, and spiritual refinement. I was taught to honor and respect the warrior way. I was told by the elders if I was to begin to live in the sacred, I must look at the behavior of all people, including myself, and understand this behavior; that could then be directed to living within the sacred.

In the late 1960s, having gone to the Lenox School in Massachusetts, I would come home to the Rosebud Reservation to spend my summers and holidays. During those times at home, I took the opportunity to talk seriously with my elder people as well as with my many relations. I recall one occasion where I was sitting discussing life with my uncle, Leo Chasing In Timber. Spontaneously, we were talking about spiritual matters. He began to tell me that there were many, many powerful medicine men in our tradition. He had known a few of them. He said that these people became holy people, not because of their visions, but because they acted in a certain way. This behavior became acknowledged as power, as strength, as expressing the will of *Tunkasila*. With care and thought, he said, "The old man, White Lance, taught me this. I will share with you what he said to me. He said, 'This gift of the Sacred Pipe is not a gift to manipulate the world, nor to manipulate others. This gift was given so that you, as a person, could start walking in a way appropriate to the needs of all, including *Tunkasila*.' White Lance said to me, 'This pipe was a gift to show Lakota people how to live, how to behave, how to prepare for the ultimate union of oneself with

53

the Spirit World. A human being has a whole lifetime to make this preparation and to perfect the journey that has to be taken.'"

Uncle Leo said, "Old man White Lance said that there are four things attached to this pipe. The first is *Wowahwala*." In Lakota this translates to calmness, stillness, tranquillity. "The second thing is *Wotakuye* (to make relations). The third thing is *Wicozani* (the well-being of all). And the fourth thing," he said, "attached to this pipe, according to old man White Lance, is *Wicouncage* (the growth and development of all things)."

I listened very carefully to Uncle Leo. He told me that old man White Lance was a very powerful healer, a visionary, and one of the strongest medicine people that he had encountered. Those words he shared were words that stuck with me. When I encountered the Sage, or the *I Ching,* the *Book of Changes,* one of the primary things I noticed in my initial study was the path of virtue that is required of the superior man who walks in balance and harmony with spirit. Of course, the Taoist tradition identifies the supreme virtue as the combination of four cardinal virtues: the first being peace, the second harmony, the third justice, and the fourth wisdom. As I realized that these four cardinal virtues were taught in the Tao as the way for man to find perfection in the development of character, I began to relate in my own mind the connection to the ways of being connected to the pipe. As told to Uncle Leo by White Lance and passed on to me, I had a direct connection between the words used in the Tao and in Lakota to describe Supreme Virtue. Peace, in Western ideology, is mostly mistaken for calmness, for tranquillity, for stillness. In Lakota, the word *Wowahwala* means that calmness, stillness. The connection I made between the two words is that in order for action to begin appropriately in its movement to peace, there must be calmness. I saw a direct correlation between the Tao of peace and in Lakota tradition, a calmness, a centeredness. Now, peace, as a definition, is the complete union of the creative energies and the receptive, birthing energies of life. In the Lakota sense of calmness, *Wowahwala* means that point before these energies unite to create the most dynamic progression in expression of life.

I was fascinated by the correlation. In Lakota, *Wotakuye,* to make relations, is connected directly to the virtue of harmony. Because harmony, as a process, presupposes a state of opposition between two forces of different nature having to unite their energies in a common direction and moving together to an achievement. I realized that the Lakota word, *Wotakuye,* to make relations, again referred directly to this process. *Wotakuye* implies making relations to harmonize the energies for unity of effort, uniting endeavor toward a common achievement. That connected deeply with me.

For the Lakota word *Wicozani,* well-being, I looked at the cardinal virtue expressed in the Tao, justice. Justice means that everything in life gets what is due it according to its nature; it gets that which constitutes its happiness without harm to anything else. If one is just, the well-being of self, the well-being of others, the well-being of all, occurs. So again, direct connection, correlation between the two thought systems was forming harmoniously.

Finally, wisdom, in the Tao, is seen as the discernment of all the laws in the universe that allow the appropriate growth and development of all things so that they will endure. In Lakota, *Wicouncage* is that which is developing and growing. For

55

instance, a generation is seen as *Wicouncage*. So, if all generations are to endure, wisdom must be the guiding force in knowing the laws that make the duration of each generation possible. So I let the two thoughts reverberate deeply in my mind as one truth. Yes! This is the way that I am being shown, not only by my people, but by the truth and wisdom of many generations. All are human experiences reaffirming this truth.

Having heard this story about what White Lance thought was connected to the behavior associated with the pipe, I began to correlate it to my own study of the wisdom being taught to me by the Sage. When I began to learn the Lakota sacred songs and had the spiritual experiences to connect these things, I understood that the truth being shown was a divine guidance directing me toward a practical way of living. The only proof of its truth is that if I live by, or attempt with my best capabilities to live by its direction, it should lead to a connection in balance with the Spirit.

The gift of the Sacred Pipe was an event in which White Buffalo Calf Woman came to the Lakota people and said, "Do it this way." The gift of the pipe was one event. After that gift was given, many holy people within the Lakota began to have visions. They began to have direction from the Spirit World in what was to be done with the pipe in practice, in ceremony, and in ritual. Stories still exist that connect certain visions to certain rituals and ceremonies that actually name people who had these visions. Since much has been written about these visions, and the ways associated from those visions with the pipe, I will not go into them here. I will simply list the seven major rituals that became attached to the Sacred Pipe. These rites were developed over a period of time after the initial gift of the pipe.

The seven rituals associated with the Sacred Pipe are first, Soul Keeping, often said in Lakota as *Wanagi Yuhapi*, "holding the ghost" or "holding the Soul." The second ritual, *Isna Ta Awica Lowanpi*, is a ritual connected to the first menstrual period of a young woman. The words translate to "singing for her menses," or "singing for her inner alone time." The third ritual relates to the puberty process. In Lakota, *Tapa Wankaya Yeyapi* literally translates into "throwing the ball up." This is a ritual showing the Lakota people that a young woman, holding the world in her hands, is now ready to be a woman, a mother. The fourth ritual is called *Hunkapi*. The literal translation comes from *Hun,* which means to cut, and *ka* (from *kan*), making a cut through that which preceded relationship. We translate it in the current Lakota as "making relations," entering into relationship, aside from the blood relationship that you were born into. And this is seen as a most sacred ritual between two individuals to hold and honor each other in sacredness, without a blood relationship.

Those first four rituals, in my own mind, are the feminine rituals of the pipe. The fifth ritual is called *Inipi*. The literal translation is "making a connection to breath," the breath of life. The figurative translation of that would be "making a connection with life." We have always understood it in the Lakota sense as purifying oneself.

The sixth ritual is called *Hanbleceyapi*, "crying in the night." Another way that Lakota people understand "crying in the night" comes from *Ceykiya*, which means "to beseech one" or "to make relation within something." And so, the elders who took me on my vision quest said that *Hanbleceya* is really to let go of yourself, so that you could find yourself in the order of all beings.

57

The seventh ritual of the Sacred Pipe, the one we consider the highest and directed at the warrior tradition, is called *Wiwayang Wacipi,* "looking at the Sun Dance." This ceremony, according to the elders who shared their thoughts with me, was seen as the turning point, the rebirth, of the warrior back into life to live again.

So, all seven of those rituals were connected to the Way of the Sacred Pipe. The rituals did not come with the pipe at the time the gift was given. But as in all traditions, when dynamic change and transformation are presented to the people, the holy people connect with and are given direction from the Spirit World to meet the needs of those times. I believe that these rituals developed out of the growth and development of the Lakota people, and the need expressed and the demands created by those changes and transformations. Many of our holy people, in connection with the Spirit World, were given ways to do this.

So the song that is used to make a connection to the Sacred Pipe and the Spirit World says, "Friend," meaning relationship or friend, "do it this way," much akin to saying, "live this way." I was also told that this song originally came from the *Tapa Wankaya Yeyapi* ceremony and went through several metamorphoses. It finally came down to the word usage in the song as it is being sung now. People understand this song in our current tradition as a pipe-filling song. It was the song, initially in its older forms, that showed the world that this young girl, becoming a woman, was now ready to be a mother. She held the world in her hands in this way. And so, I see a connection between this song and the teaching of holding the world in your hands. If you can birth new being, new living into this world, you are truly connected to the Sacred.

58

What I have learned in the song and the message that it contains for me is a way of being. It gives the message that shows how one should conduct oneself at the beginning of anything, whether it be into the sacred, or whether it be into living within your world and its relationships. There is an appropriate behavior to act within. Since our Lakota culture, still, is largely defined as a warrior culture, the teachings of the old people showed me a way to look at the warrior tradition and also a way to look at the sacred tradition.

I had an uncle who became a grandfather of mine by marriage (he married my Uncle Leo's mother, Lena Eagle Man). His name was Charlie Black Bear. Charlie was a very interesting individual who loved to dance. He used to attend *Wacipis* and get dressed even if no one else did. When he heard the music, he would put the bells and his outfit on. He would go out into the dance ground and just be in a state of exhilaration and enthusiasm. Moving in rhythm to the beat of the drum, he enjoyed the music being performed by a group of singers. In our times together, we were sent out often to go pick currants, chokecherries, plums, juneberries, and occasionally, to go dig what we called *Tinpsila,* which is the wild turnip. We would have axes, buckets, or shovels on many of our excursions. Whenever I stayed with my Uncle Leo and Christina, Charlie would wake me up early in the morning. He would say, "*Takoja* (Grandson, or grandchild)! *Hiyuwo* (Come on)! Let's go get a turnip today." Or "Let's go get some plums today." Because we rarely rode horseback or wagons for these journeys, we would always walk and enjoy the nature around us. It was always a time for him to talk with me.

Once when we went to dig *Tinpsila* (wild turnip), he said seriously, "Our people used to have strange relationships with

59

other tribes." Pausing, taking a breath, he continued, "I knew a man by the name of Bear In The Woods. He told me a story. He left here riding a horse to go up north, past White River. As he was coming down toward the river, there near White River, he saw a small group of men who were on what he thought was a *Zuyapi* (war party or adventure). He knew he was in trouble when he saw these young men coming after him." That's one of the traditions of the warriors; they're always picking on each other at opportune times. He said, "This Bear In The Woods realized he had stumbled onto a very aggressive group of young men. He wasn't quite sure whether they were Arikawa, or Pawnee (they were the same people), or Kiowa, or other men; he didn't have time to notice. But he could see their aggression. So he started to ride back away from the river at full gallop. Out of a ravine came this young man who tried to jump in front of the horse that Bear In The Woods was riding. Bear In The Woods took his knife, and he swooped down in a motion toward the young warrior who was jumping in his way. He cut him from below the ribcage all the way across, up to his shoulder. Bear In The Woods, when he saw that he did this, kept riding. He was sure that that warrior was dead, but he kept riding, leaving the scene." Grandpa Charlie asked me, "What do you think about that?"

I said to Grandpa Charlie, "Sounds like those war parties and those times were dangerous."

And he said, "Yeah, but think about this. Bear In The Woods told me that story. He told me to think about it." He said, "You think about this—what do you think?"

As we kept walking, he grinned at me. "I have another story. I knew an old man. I forget his name now, but he was related to the Thin Elks up north of here, up toward Ring

Thunder. He had relations down this way toward the Owl Bonnet community. And so, this old man," he said, "he woke up one morning and took his grandson out into the woods. This old man decided to teach his grandson how to make a true bow and arrow, not a toy, but a true bow and arrow. He began to teach him the whole thing; how you cut the wood, how you dry it, how you take animal hide and get sinew, and how you create a tension for the bow so it has great strength and great ability to send an arrow far. How to kill game. And he made him some arrows with stone heads. He made this to show his grandson how to do this, taking time to do it. He made a bow that was very, very strong and powerful. One day he was in his tent and he heard his grandson saying, 'Grandpa, come out! I want to show you something!' And so, the old man came rushing out of the tent. Outside, the young boy said to him, 'See, I can shoot this!' He pointed the bow and arrow at his grandfather. He pulled the tightness of the sinew, and he let the arrow fly. The arrow entered the old man's eye and went up into his head. And the old man expressed pain and said to his grandson, 'What have you done to me?' "

Grandpa Charlie paused, then said, "The old man didn't die right then. He suffered a little bit before he died, but he passed away. And I remember this!" He looked at me intently. "What do you think of this? What do you think of what the little boy did to that old man?"

Of course, now I had two stories. We were still walking, trying to find the turnips. One thing about turnips, they don't jump out in front of you. You have to find them. So we were looking on the prairie floor to see where these turnips might be growing.

61

As we were looking, I thought about the stories. I asked him, "Grandpa Charlie, really, what are you trying to tell me?"

He said, "*Takoja* (grandson), do we really ever know what is really good and what is really bad? That young warrior, Bear In The Woods, if he killed someone like that in today's world, he would be put behind those iron bars. He would be considered an evil man. In his time, what he did was part of surviving, part of living." He said, "Is what he did evil? Really bad?" He said, "Look at the little grandson. Did he have an intent to kill his grandfather? Or was he playing a game where he could show his grandfather that he learned how to use this bow? And what did his grandfather teach him about using this bow?" He said, "Is that an evil, what that little boy did? Is that an evil what the grandfather did, to put a weapon into a young boy's hands? Don't you think that we really need to sit sometimes, look at our world, and see what is really good in it and what is really evil in it?" He said, "These are occasions where I have been told stories that made me think about these things. What is really good, and what is really bad? *Takoja,* think about these things."

I realized that he cautioned me through other stories he told me about warriors and how life was on the plains. He said, "It's not very good sometimes to look backward toward the past thinking that we had a better life back then. It is better always to look at what you are doing today to make the determination of whether life is good or not."

There were several occasions where Grandma Lena, Grandpa Charlie's wife, would sit down and tell me, "*Takoja* (grandson), don't think of the past as being better than what we have now, no matter how difficult life gets. I want to show you something." We would go outside and she'd say, "See that toilet out there?" (The toilets we used back in those days were outhouses.) You go in there and you have magazines, newspapers, and sometimes toilet paper to use to wipe your butt with." (My ears burned because I was listening to this grandmother of mine use words like that!) She went on, "In the old days, we didn't have newspapers, magazines, and toilet paper. These are luxuries of our time. In the old days, if you didn't wipe your butt, you stunk! And there were many people walking around these plains who would stink. If you had to go to the bathroom, you didn't go to an outhouse. You had the open plains, so you went behind bushes or trees, away from camp to do this! And you did not always have the luxury of cleanliness. Now what is good about that in the past?" she would ask.

So I kept that in mind. From these little stories, what I learned was that in the warrior tradition or in any effort that a human being makes, the first step taken is always a step of moving back toward harmony, togetherness in behavior, with your relations in this world. I learned that directly from my many grandparents; to even begin to move to achievement, to finish anything, requires you to look at how you do things, what you do, and how what you do relates to your world.

Patterns began to emerge from those stories that the elders taught me that really showed me something. First of all, if you as a person, warrior or not, decide that you want to embark on a journey or set a goal to complete, or just move to work with other people for a common purpose, the first step that you must take is to truly look at what you do, if only to see the possibility of accomplishing that which you set in the first place. So, the

63

patterns that I saw in the stories shared with me directed me to begin to look at what was real in all things, in all the ways I could.

When we begin to look at how we behave in relation to others, we begin to realize that everything is related to each other in some form or fashion. Many grandfathers and grandmothers said to me, "That's why we say, *Mitakuye oyas'in,* in our prayers and in our acknowledgment of all that is truly related."

The warriors who that day encountered the White Buffalo Calf Woman had a goal. They had a mission. That mission was to go and find nourishment for the people. When they encountered White Buffalo Calf Woman, there was a difference of approach by the two warriors toward the sacred event of encountering her.

When the old people talked about the challenge of uniting people (a common theme in Lakota tradition), the problem was always addressed in terms of finding a way to nourish the people so that they could unite their wills and achieve a common purpose successfully. Much of ritual and ceremony among the Lakota was specifically designed to unite the minds and the will of the people toward a common purpose.

When the elders talked about how one begins the spiritual journey, they always thought the young people had the most difficult time beginning their journey toward balance and toward harmony. In terms of the human condition, the elders often talked about the young people as being wild and extremely difficult to influence. In our talks, they talked about approaching the young people with good behavior even when the young ones became irritable and angry.

When Grandpa Charlie and Grandma Lena used to tease me about looking to the old ways as better or purer than how we were living, they and some other elders I encountered along the way tried to teach me a truth about our nature. Life is simply an expression of nature. When people find out who they are, what they should do with who they are, and that what they do in life corresponds with what they bring to the world with their own capabilities and inner worth, they are expressing their nature. When they do this, they find their appropriate place in relation to their world. Once done, the elders felt that order and agreement reigned in the tribe.

They would always tell me that when we begin something, right at the beginning everything is simple and so our conduct, our behavior, in its simplicity remains free of any social obligations. We are somewhat free to follow our wishes and our desires in contentment and no trouble occurred if we made no demands on people. Every individual who begins a journey of some kind, a mission, a goal, a spiritual quest, that simple position is a very weak position at the start. So that person must draw on inner strength that can move one forward. At the same time, one has to learn to be content with simplicity in that forward movement, so that no fault is incurred in relation to others.

The old people used to say that when a person becomes dissatisfied with modest circumstances, that person becomes restless, ambitious, and tries to force forward movement. Usually, not for the sake of accomplishing anything worthwhile, but mainly to get away from what that person perceives as lowliness, inferiority, or poverty. And of course, from that perspective, if that person achieves what they are after, it usually leads to arrogance and isolation from others. And so, that person has made a mistake.

But likewise, the old people felt that a person who becomes good at what they offer to the world and what their

65

inner worth shows they can do in the world becomes very content with simplicity and behaves in that way. So, the wish to move forward is the wish to accomplish something that is good, something that is worthwhile. When this kind of person attains that goal in doing something worthwhile, everything becomes as it should be. But that person also still must be very careful in that progress forward because anything that is worthwhile encounters conflict at the beginning. A person who is not strong within will become very deceptive, and will use guile and cunning to try to achieve their purpose. A person with deep cunning, who has a fixed determination to get their way, also becomes extremely quarrelsome and confrontational.

66

The old people said that a person who knows how to look at what doesn't work, what doesn't unite, and knows how to deal with conflict, especially when correctness and opposition is present, has to realize that nothing great can be accomplished in conflict. Anything that can be accomplished in a worthwhile manner or successfully requires a unity and harmony of forces. Among people, a great need is created to have a unified purpose, a unified mind. When a union has conflict within, there is no power to deal with danger that comes from without. And the old people felt that the best way to handle conflict was to realize that when one begins anything, one is in a position to see what doesn't work and also to see what does work.

To avoid conflict, the old people felt that everything had to be truly looked at very carefully right at the beginning. And a person has to determine what rights one has and what has to be accomplished to make certain that the spiritual trends of all people in a goal or movement forward harmonize. If this harmonization exists, conflict is removed right at the beginning.

In the community where I spent most of my youth, especially in my teen years, there was a man named Charlie Turning Bear. When I knew him he was well into his sixties. Many people had great respect for him because he knew some of the old ways and was active in community endeavors and activities. He had a bad case of arthritis, so he could barely get around, but he walked everywhere. And my grandfathers and my grandmothers and my aunts and uncles had a very humorous and affectionate relationship with the man. Most of the people believed that he was wise. He was very centered in his own ways, but without aggression toward anyone. He appeared to withdraw from the hurries of life, seemed to seek nothing, rarely asked anything of anyone, and wasn't seduced or enticed into anything that did not seem right. And he appeared to be very true to himself, and even toward the end of his life seemed to be very much on the level road. What I saw in him was a contentment and an acceptance of fate. And so he seemed to be very free of entanglements. His relatives looked at him as a person who appeared very much alone, maybe even lonely. But they also had a great respect for him because he seemed to walk a very smooth and level road.

Some of the comments people made when speaking of him were that he was an individual who worked very hard to purify himself toward the end of his days. He, like many other human beings, certainly had times when he made mistakes, as well as times of challenge. But all of my relations looked at him as a person who honored his own goodness and allowed his goodness to guide him in all of his activities. He seemed to be devoted to the Spirit within himself, and so it appeared that he was attaining a great degree of innocence. And at least a majority of the time, he appeared to be doing correct things, right things, with confidence and without any thought of reward or personal advantage. And he even passed away by himself in his cabin.

By the time he passed away, many people had watched him live out his life in ways that were certainly his own to live. And he had great respect from many because they thought that he was right in what he was doing, and he was certainly connecting with the will of *Tunkasila*. And my grandmother used to say to me, "Look at him, and if you ever find yourself alone, maybe you ought to follow his example."

Then she would say, "If a person doesn't purify himself, *Tunkasila* and the *Wakan Oyate,* the spirit people, do not bless his actions." So I learned from that that we have to learn how to draw on the spiritual wealth that is within us, that we really truly do have command of. That spiritual wealth is also around us, expressing itself through the life that we share in this time, in this world. If we know how to draw on this spiritual wealth, we can take care to relate properly to all forms of life, to all forms of doing things, and to be able to lend a hand, lend help, to further these things toward the good with proper timing.

Charlie Turning Bear was not the only person that I was asked to look at as an example. I learned to look at my own world with the realization that one has to learn to do everything that has to be accomplished for its own sake, as the time and place demand. Also, I learned that I should not get caught up with how perfect the result should be, but I should do what has to be done. And when whatever is necessary is done appropriately, everything turns out well. What we do becomes accomplished in a worthwhile manner.

68

Relating back to the warriors, they had to learn how to find game and how to be able to take it, so that they could bring what they had accomplished back to the people for their nourishment.

Another grandfather, my maternal grandfather, Robert Little Hawk, talked to me about the warrior way. He was involved in one of the world wars, as a soldier. He thought that a warrior who got caught up in his own strength, in his own wishes and desires, and who wanted the world his way without looking at his relationships appropriately, always exposed himself to dangerous situations and invited evil consequences or disaster, because he was taking on something that was beyond his abilities and strength. He thought warriors of this kind were reckless. They moved ahead without thought, without caution, and without care.

He said that these warriors who did this were inadequate to express their true power in an appropriate way. The only good that these warriors could do, he used to say, is to have a worthwhile cause to die for. Warriors of this nature already had given up their lives because they were looking at the world with one eye. They were walking with lameness. Grandpa thought that that was not a very wise way for a warrior to be.

A warrior who truly wants to do that which is right, he used to say, is helped by creation; he's helped by the universe. A warrior, because he sits on the edge of life and death, had to learn how to make himself strong, tireless. But he said that the warrior eventually had to leave the warrior way behind in order to connect to the Spirit World. In order for the warrior who does things right to live a long time, he had to learn how to find the greatest goodness in himself, so that whatever he left behind would last.

69

Grandpa Robert used to take me along on many activities, such as going for wood, chopping wood, hunting rabbits and
prairie dogs to eat, as well as picking berries, chokecherries, and
plums—like my other grandfathers. He worked effortlessly to
convince me that a person had to work to make himself strong
in every way. He said we had to understand what is good and
what is really bad. We have to throw out, with clear thinking, all
that is weak, all that is degrading, and all that is bad, to be the
best that we can. He was convinced that it was the only way to
gain energy. You gain energy because you limit your actions to
those which you know you can accomplish.

Another grandfather of mine used to tell me that any person, man or woman, had to learn how to persist in whatever they
started. And he used to say that if you work for someone, you
must learn how to finish the work that you are given without
trying to be better than the person that you are working for.
What that showed me was that we have to learn how to free ourselves of vanity. We have to understand our abilities so that we
do not attract attention in such a way that we are put in a position where we are directed to do something that we cannot do.
Even in relation to a large group of people, if we are working on
finding out who and what we are, it should be done with a certain degree of restraint. Best not to seek fame, or the public eye.

Grandpa Robert was of the mind that it would be better
to finish those things you know you can, so that you send energy
and forces into motion that can later accomplish something truly
worthwhile. So he used to say, "Learn to finish your work in such
a way that it gives you other opportunities. And that way, you
don't throw yourself away, and you also don't put yourself in a

position where you gain a way that is manipulated by the people. One of the great dangers for anyone, and we used to see this among the warriors," he would say, "is when a person's fame begins to spread outward, all the people run to this person. They consider this person a hero. And usually this happens because he or she shows adequacy in that which is presented to be accomplished. And when there's all sorts of things to be done, this kind of person jumps into all kinds of activity, all kinds of plans, and worries begin to press in. It's as though this person comes out of darkness into bright light, and everybody wants this person to do something for them. So, many times a warrior is ruined by what the people demand of him or her because the people pulled him into their course." And he used to use a word that I can now perhaps translate as ambition. He said, "Ambition, the want to do things with your abilities beyond your time to do them, destroys your integrity, your goodness of being. A person with ambition forgets that true greatness is not tempted by fame or by personal gain. If a warrior knows how to meet the demands that people place on him, he can be cautious enough to avoid failure without making mistakes." So I learned that the beginning of anything is very important in one's journey, in one's movement forward.

A person with caution and with great clarity can do dangerous things. The old people used to say that people who are clear or cautious, who can look at a situation from many different ways, can do the most dangerous things because they are applying inner capabilities and strengths in a correct manner.

One must really be careful about what one is pulled in to do, or wishes to do. If one has confidence to accomplish

71

something worthwhile to achieve one's purpose, caution, along with the right attitude and with the right ability, will always overcome danger in that progress forward.

This is because the person of this ability can, with caution, truly learn how to deal with the world and the relationships in it. A person of this nature knows how to deal with people who are difficult to influence. This type of person knows how to connect with people, understand, and gain great influence over others when one acts within the truth of one's own being. A person who acts with this kind of truth knows that simple bonds with people can turn very quickly into hatred because of competition or personal ambition. When common interests between people cease, the union that was agreed to begins to cease.

Grandpa used to say, "Those who are very close friends, who are competitive with each other, can end up hating each other. So when you work with others, this friendship has to be right. One has to be so committed to that friendship that it can be strong in overcoming anything. But one has to learn how to remove holding judgment in any kind of situation. We must learn to understand human beings, to understand life. We have to sympathize and appreciate all circumstances that we're in. And if you know how to forgive someone, and pardon them their mistakes, you are showing a true strength, and you get many who respect it and who will work with you. This kind of strength knows very little weakness.

"So it's important," he would say, "that we learn to put all of our desires, all of our feelings, and all of our passions and wants in the right place, not to have things the way we want them, but to learn how any situation, any group of people, anything that you do, shows what is needed to achieve anything worthwhile."

My Grandma Mary used to say that we should never become so stuck on something that we do not see what is around us. There are some things in life that require you to be firm, to be determined, but you have to learn that being strong and determined when you are walking this way for a time can get you stuck, and such "stuckness" can become very dangerous. You look at the road ahead of you and all you see is where you are going. You forget the beauty of all that exists on each side of that road. So, she used to say, "When people are estranged from each other and they disagree, it is important for them to learn what the disagreement is about and to determine if that disagreement can be overcome. Everything we do requires other people in it to finish to make it worthwhile." She said, "When you get into relationships with others, look at your viewpoints, look at what you see, and make certain that they move in the same direction. If they go too far widely from each other, very little can be accomplished. And if you are in a situation where there is disagreement, difference of view, difference of thought, but you know you can come together, learn how to hold yourself to doing those things that you know you can get done, because you know that the relationship you have, your friendship, can come to agreement at some point. So we do have to accept in life some things that are opposite that have to learn how to work together. And when that's accomplished," she would say, "everything takes its right place." She said, "But in order to arrive at that right place, you have to honor who you are. Don't get pulled into vulgar things. Avoid being pulled into weak things. Especially when you are working with other people. Learn how to be yourself. Preserve who you are." And of course, that made sense.

When my blood brother Joe was killed in a car accident in 1969, Grandpa Sam Bear was one of the elders who sat me down and gave me a long lecture because I was so angry, so upset, so hurt. And I remember distinctly only a few lines that he voiced to me that day. He took me aside and said, "All of us human beings have a day that is meant for us to go back to where we came from. On some occasions that day can be known, but most of the time we don't know when the day is that is our time to reconnect with Spirit, to leave this body that you hold behind and go back to the Spirit World, which is the real world." He said, "You must learn how to regain some happiness, some joy in your life. This anger and this pain you hold will pass one day. You'll always remember your brother, but you must remember there's a part of you that has to keep living because this gift of life comes from a greater source than you or I. You can always draw on this source. Look at what you've done. Look at the good things that you have accomplished. Look at the good things that your brother is leaving for you in the short time you've spent together. When everything is seen in the way of that which has been accomplished," he said, "we know that goodness prevails. Our action and what that action produces in the world will tell you whether there's a good life for you ahead or whether there's a shorter life ahead for you. So look at what you must do that is good and you'll make certain that you'll begin to live a good life.

"No one really knows oneself. The part that belongs to *Tunkasila* is a part you'll never know, you can only allow it to work through you, but in this world it's only by what you have done, those things you've accomplished, that you can look at and know what to expect. So from this time forward, learn to let your brother go, learn to get ahold of yourself, and start doing good things. In this way you can expect the good to prevail in your life." And, because alcohol was involved in the accident that killed my brother, he said, "But it's important in this happiness to look at what your brother has left you. You don't want to do the same thing. If you get caught up in all the pleasures of this world, all the seductions of this world, if you get caught up in them you begin to be unstable. And the pleasures of this world that you don't leave aside or leave alone begin to have so powerful an influence and effect in your life that you're pulled along by them. When this occurs, look at your brother: an accident such as this happens. We call this accident, but a pleasure of the world has cost his life. When you give up direction of your life, what happens to you becomes unknowable. Chance in all those things around you begin to take your life. So learn how to be strong, to be solid. But in the world, learn to go with the flow of things. Learn how to adapt to those things. Be gentle. This kind of happiness affects everything around you in a good way. Be strong. Be honest with yourself. This kind of thinking toward *Tunkasila, Wakantanka,* and others allows you to achieve good things. So let your brother go."

He sat down beside me and cried. His kind display of care took me out of the real deep anger I was feeling. And it made me look at death not as a dynamic force of life but just as a doorway to another place. Because of the talk given to me by Grandpa Sam, I felt allowed to look at happiness and joy instead,

75

and I began to cry more for the happy times that I had experienced with my brother.

Grandpa Sam's talk also allowed me to rejoin my friends and to not get caught up in the grief that was so deep in me. And that particular event with Grandpa Sam also taught me that I had to still respect the life around me, which included my relations, my other brothers, my grandmothers, my grandfathers, aunts and uncles, father, mother, and the little ones whom I was beginning to see come into the world at that time. I began to see light again. Also, for me, the spiritual phrase, "*Kola, lecel ecun wo* (Friend, do it this way)!" was beginning to have meaning.

4

Look Upon This Pipe,
It Is Sacred!

Wayankeye yo!	Look upon it!
Wayankeye yo!	Look upon it!
Wayankeye!	Look!
Canunpa ki le,	This Pipe,
Wakan yelo!	Is sacred!
Wayankeye yo!	Look upon it!
Wayankeye yo!	Look upon it!
Ocokan ki le,	This center place,
Wakan yelo!	Is sacred!
Wayankeye yo!	Look upon it!
Wayankeye yo!	Look upon it!
Wiyaka ki le,	This feather,
Wakan yelo!	Is sacred!
Wayankeye yo!	Look upon it!

This song is sung after the *Canunpa* has been filled with tobacco, and the spiritual leader is offering it to the *Wakan Oyate,* the Spirit People.

I was told by some of the spiritual elders and ceremonial leaders what this song referred to. In Lakota, *Wayankayo* means to perceive, to look upon. In the song, we notice that we are pointing to the Pipe as sacred. In the center, the altar is sacred. When you are singing to the Spirit World, and you are defining something as sacred, singing the sacred language, the Spirit is speaking to you, and you in turn are speaking to the Spirit. So the process becomes one of reaching an agreement of what is considered sacred. You are making something sacred. And so, *Wayanka yo,* look upon, goes beyond the meaning of seeing with one's eyes. It means to make an appearance of that which is defined in this song as sacred.

On one of our journeys to go pick plums, Grandpa Charlie Black Bear said some things to me which were very interesting. We grabbed a couple of pails from the house and he said, "Let's go pick some plums!" We started out early in the morning going west of the house where he lived. It was late June. The morning was clear. Meadowlarks were out. You could hear all kinds of birds singing their songs. It seemed to me like a good day to go pick some berries instead (since we were in the first green of the plums for that time of the year).

Usually, when Grandpa Charlie and I went out, we would look for the place that had the most plums and berries, so it would make the job easier. So walking west of the house in Two Strike Community, we were headed down toward the Little White River, which is about six miles west of Two Strike. As we were walking over the crest of a hill, I noticed that there was a quick buildup of thunder clouds. By the time we were going down toward the river, the thunder clouds were overhead. It started to sprinkle rain.

Grandpa Charlie looked up and said, "This must be a good day! We're being washed by the *Wakinyan* (Thunder Beings). There must be a good message in that." When you hear this in Lakota, you immediately conjure up in your mind pictures of beings and actual three-dimensional pictures of things that the other person is talking to you about. So I was, in my mind, thinking what the *Wakinyan* were doing up in the clouds; I was thinking they were throwing water on us. And it felt good in that we seemed to be the only ones receiving this water.

Grandpa said, "*Takoja,* the *Wakinyan* carry this gift of life, this water. Life in our world can't exist without it. So when it rains like this, you should always thank *Wakan Tanka,* the Great Spirit. The Great Spirit, *Wakan Tanka,* uses the *Wakinyan,* Thunder Beings, to give nourishment to the plant people and to us." He said, "This sun comes up in the east every morning and it goes down, drops in the west in the evening. And nighttime comes. So this water that's falling here, it wears away at these hills that you and I are walking. It takes the earth off these hills, and carries it down to the river. And the river carries this dirt many, many miles filling up the low places. And this night sun, the moon, it's dark a good portion of the time. And it's light a good portion of the time. It balances itself in this light and this darkness. Anything that has fullness begins to lose its fullness when it becomes a situation where it cannot be full any more. So what is full, when it is really full, starts to empty itself. We are going

79

to go get plums to fill ourselves." (I still thought berries were a better choice.) "That's really preparing us for a time when we won't have it to fill ourselves. We walk this road. Every man, every woman, walks a road of experiences that becomes a full-ness of what that life is meant to be. *Wakan Tanka* makes certain that life is full, and that life is also empty."

He said, "Every man and every woman is given this will, *Wowacin,*" he called it, "to make that road be what it's supposed to be. What every man, every woman does, comes under an energy of that which is good or an energy of that which is bad. What you do when you act determines whether good comes to you, or whether bad comes to you."

He continued, "What every man or woman is learning while walking this road is to carry out the work that they're meant to do, simply because it has to be done. It doesn't make sense to brag about what's done or to honor oneself for what's been done. It's important that every man and woman simply do what has to be done. In that way, we can all learn to do good things and to love each other. Maybe that's what the *Wakinyan,* in washing us, is showing us this day." I listened. I have had many journeys with Grandpa Charlie talking about spiritual things out of his own experience. What he said was quite interesting to me. I put a little thought, but not much understanding, into what he was saying.

During the spring break of 1967, I came back to Rosebud, leaving Lenox School to take a two-week break. I was accus-tomed to sitting with my Grandma Mary after I woke up each day, and we would talk about many different things. In Lakota,. you have great freedom to talk about a lot of things. On this par-

80

ℒ♥

ticular occasion, I was asking Grandma about a certain Lakota word which is put at the end of words, to give them a meaning of the most or the ultimate. The word ending is spelled *hci*. When you put that at the end of a word, the word becomes "the most" or "the highest of anything." And so, I was trying to get her to define that in English. She was having a difficult time finding a word in English to describe the "most or the ultimate." I was amused by her efforts because she was describing to me what the word meant in Lakota. She would describe it as when you do something, and you cannot do it anymore, but it is the best or the highest of something that you do—that is what *hci* means.

I was amused, and as I was leaving to go to visit my friends, she said, "Be careful and humble yourself." Well, throughout my youth growing up with her, that was a common phrase that she would say to me. She would say, "Be careful" and "Humble yourself." Looking back, I realized that that was one of her simplest and greatest teachings to me.

Humbling yourself is a step that you take in ceremony when you say to the Spirit that you are recognizing something as sacred, the closest relationship that you have to something. And in the song, the Spirit World is saying, "Yes, this is sacred." In a song, when you address the Pipe you are addressing a way of being, a way of doing. When you address an altar, it is a place where you stop all other activity to make a connection in an appropriate manner to balance the relationship between the Spirit World and the material world.

So, throughout the years, especially after my grandmother passed away, I thought much of what she meant when she said "Be careful. Humble yourself." The Lakota words, actually, in

81

translation can mean "pity yourself, humble yourself." Another translation of the words that she used would translate to "love yourself." When I began to think of what she meant by "humble yourself," I recalled the many times she would say those words in relation to something that I would contemplate doing or was doing, or had done already. I began to form an understanding that what she was telling me was to balance my world, my activity. Balance those things that could lead me to trouble, balance those things where I would not do anything that was good. So, I began to understand that in her simple words, she was telling me to reduce that which was too much. Strengthen and enhance that which was too little. She was asking me to be cautious, balance things, make them equal. And what she was saying to me was, "Do not get caught up in any extremes." That was her simple, great lesson to me.

82

Recalling my times with Grandpa Charlie, I began to understand what he was saying, also in Lakota. In life we have to do that which is natural; we must have appropriate relationships. And in these appropriate relationships, we must know what relates to each other, so that those things that are high and those things that are low begin to complement each other. It may take a long time to achieve that balance, but if that balance is achieved it always seems easy because it becomes self-evident. So, what I was being told by both my Grandpa Charlie and my Grandma Mary was we must establish order in the world. We have to know what we consider sacred, what we consider mundane, and begin to balance the two. We must equalize those extremes, so that balance and equitable conditions occur. In doing this, we avoid discontent, discouragement, and aggression.

But, in thinking that way, I began to realize, also from my grandma's teaching, that even modesty and humility require us to be balanced. When we begin anything, or try to accomplish something, things that we have to do are easy if we know how to do them quickly and simply. Maybe it is because we learn not to impose our wishes, desires, demands, or conditions on that which we are about to finish and accomplish. We learn simply and easily, and as quickly as possible, to do what we have to do. If we do not think about it much, we do not resist that which we have to accomplish. We learn to do this equalizing, this balancing, by staying as calm as possible in any given situation. You can only do that if you exercise caution and humility as you go into any action or endeavor. When you have this calmness, even surprises and shocks only make you realize that there must be a balance between the sacred and the mundane. A shock can shake your inner calmness, but if you are truly calm, the shock or surprise only bounces off, because you have an understanding of the sacred and the mundane, that they are in relationship, and things will be done easily and simply.

We have to be careful that being humble is only expressed in our actions, in how we behave. Grandma would always point out to me that if you humble yourself, which is loving yourself, you learn to honor things as they are without illusion. What leads you to honor is truth itself. You hold that above all other considerations and all other things. Being humble requires one to balance that humility itself in relation to action. If you encounter a situation where quick action will get you out of any obstruction or danger, you simply do it because it has to be done. But the great lesson, in Grandma's words, was always that you carry things to conclusion simply because things have to be done that way.

Humility requires one to love oneself, to respect oneself. If you humble yourself, this love of yourself extends from you, and the respect generated by this love extends from you to all other beings around you. It is not a position, in being humble, to boast about the great actions you can take to finish things. But it puts you in a position to make yourself beloved and win support from those around you when you carry actions to their conclusion so that other things can be done from that point onward.

Grandma, in saying "Be careful" and "Humble yourself," was also really saying to hold proper measure in everything that you do. "If you love yourself," she used to say, "You'll do what's good for you. You'll do what is right for you." And she would be gently emphatic in her statement, "Know how to humble yourself!" which carried a warning in it.

In being confident, one can do great things. In being confident, you know how to relate properly to your relationships, where you do not abuse nor try to overcome the worth of others. She gave me a warning about false humility, "We can hide behind a cause. We can hide behind a position. We can hold a title or a position without ever being responsible. We can be paid for doing something without giving the proper work and do empty actions that don't accomplish anything." So by her saying, "Be careful and humble yourself," in many ways, she was telling me to show interest in my own life and in the work I could accomplish.

"There are times," she would say, "in which we have to do something with great force, not aggressively, but with great energy. Some things in life require energetic action for their accomplishment. In order to finish anything with great action, great energy, make sure that you have people around you who think the same way you do. Otherwise, you'll find yourself in great trouble! On the other hand, if you're certain of the people around you, and you run into great trouble, friends will come to support you. So it's important that you treat a situation for what it is. Take care not to offend anyone, especially yourself. And even in those energetic times, hold yourself humbly!"

She would lower her voice, but with firm determination look at me, and say, "If you truly are humble, it will show in your world, in your reality. It's probably best to put great effort into this, to do things simply because they have to be done without trying to convince the world that you have done it. It's enough to accomplish those things that need to be accomplished. If you fail at this, you are going to blame other people for that failure. And if others blame you for their failures, if you're not humble, you'll feel sorry for yourself, thinking that you're humble. That will keep you from defending yourself."

She said, "If you're humble, if you love yourself, you'll try to put things in order. You'll try to put things in the right place, and you'll keep your anger and your blame of others in the right place. The person you always have to watch out for is yourself. And if you want to do things correctly, love yourself and learn how to be still. If you're still, keep your mind clear and you'll avoid mistakes."

It took me a long time to realize that she was teaching me a great lesson about life in its extremes. How I should handle them. In coming to agreement with others, and especially the

85

Spirit World, we must know what we consider sacred and what we agree to as being sacred. To consider the Sacred Pipe is to take on a walk of life that at the beginning looks at harmonizing and balancing so that things can be set in order. We can accomplish great things. That was her lesson to me.

In our ceremony, by singing this song, we are now acknowledging that our walk, that our talk, is now going into the sacred. We must begin to think in terms of having a proper relationship with that which is sacred.

5

To the Four Directions
I Am Related

Kola!	Friend!
Howaye lo!	I send my voice!
Kola!	Friend!
Howaye lo!	I send my voice!
Wiohpeyata,	At the west,
Sunka Wakan Oyate wan,	A Horse Nation,
Sitomniya,	Everywhere,
Taku yayin kte lo!	You will make relations!
Ehapi k'un?	(Remember) you said this?
Howaye lo!	I send my voice!
Kola!	Friend!
Howaye lo!	I send my voice!
Waziyata,	At the north,
Tatanka Oyate wan,	A Buffalo Nation,

Sitomniya,	Everywhere,
Taku yayin kte lo!	You will make relations!
Ehapi k'un?	(Remember) you said this?
Howaye lo!	I send my voice!
Kola!	Friend!
Howaye lo!	I send my voice!
Wiohenyanpata,	At the east,
Hehaka Oyate wan,	An Elk Nation,
Sitomniya,	Everywhere,
Taku yayin kte lo!	You will make relations!
Ehapi k'un?	(Remember) you said this?
Howaye lo!	I send my voice!
Kola!	Friend!
Howaye lo!	I send my voice!
Itokagata,	At the south,
Wamakaskan Oyate wan,	A Plant Nation,
Sitomniya,	Everywhere,
Taku yayin kte lo!	You will make relations!
Ehapi k'un?	(Remember) you said this?
Howaye lo!	I send my voice!
Kola! ·	Friend!
Howaye lo!	I send my voice!

88

There are numerous variations and songs that are called *Tatioye Topa Olowan* (Four Directions Songs). I have chosen this song for the purposes of our ceremony. I have even excluded the most sacred Four Directions Song that others sing for the *Lowanpi*. I wanted to show that for the holy man to begin to make a connection to the Spirit World, he must begin to make a connection with all of his *Wotakuyepi* (relations), and this song gives an inkling of what that is. All Four Directions Songs have language that begins to connect the whole Universe to this ceremonial process. I have just chosen one of many for our ceremony.

When we sing the Four Directions Song, the song acknowledges all the directions (above and below are also included in some songs). In this song, we are asking for a recognition of one's own being in the wholeness of the sacred. But the Spirit is also acknowledging through the song its own sacredness to the relationship that is being asked for. This in turn creates a turning point or return to goodness in the life that is being expressed.

In recognizing that we are a center of an experience, we must also recognize that we share a reality that has other centers with their own realities and experiences. We must conclude at some point in our lives that there must be a common divine reality that belongs to every living thing upon the earth. When we begin to recognize this universe and world of relationships, a return to the understanding, acceptance, and recognition of this great force of life occurs. We can call it the good. We can call it the love. We can call it the light. Regardless of what we call it, this movement back to what is natural begins to arise spontaneously. In recognition of this relationship to all things, we move easily beyond the old. Recognizing it puts us in a position to discard the old and open ourselves to what is new in the Spirit and material worlds. It is an acknowledgment to move away from the harm and injuries of the old, and open ourselves to the regeneration and the rising of the new.

In ceremony, to a large extent, we are in a circle of people who share the same views. If the others in the ceremony do not have the same views, one purpose of the ceremony is to form a common view, a common focus. When we agree to come into the ceremony, we harmonize ourselves and our beings to this time; we are taking a step in which we must put all selfish tendencies aside. At the least, we must act on the inclination to put mistakes or wrongs aside. If what we are doing is correct, we find that we do not need to rush anything artificially or by desire. This common mind, this common focus, begins to unfold itself in a timely manner. When we acknowledge that we are at the center of relationship, but also that we are at the outside of other centers of relationship, we see that which is within and that which is without. Through the ceremony, we begin to connect with life energy when we recognize our relationship to all that is.

The movement that we make through this song is at the beginning of the ceremony, so we enter this ceremony slowly, almost resting. We do this so that we will not dissipate what we are building. Through the song, we treat the time with caution, with care, with tenderness, so that this return to spirit can lead to a flowering.

In life, what we learn in making proper relationships and acknowledging proper relationships is that we can return to a good path no matter what wrongs we may have committed, or what inappropriate decisions and actions have led us to in consequence. If we have the will to correct mistakes and experience goodness, we can only correct mistakes when we know that we have only slightly fallen off the path of goodness and righteousness. We can always turn back to that which is good before we go too far in doing wrong.

In learning how to reconnect with the sacred and to have faith in it, we learn to grow appropriately in goodness and in the proper relationship. So in mind, before we would go into a ceremony or an *Inipi,* the elders would say, "Put all that is negative, put all that is even faintly bad aside immediately. Don't let it take root in your thought. Don't let it get that far." In this way you make certain that all will go well. There will be no reason to feel sorry for anything.

All the things that are seen as bad in the outcomes of human activity cannot just happen; they take time to develop. If you think you can get away with little wrongs, little faults, your indifference to accepting the bad qualities of these things will in time cause you to make a great mistake. They will lead you to a great fall, because you do not treat the weak and the inappropriate as the very things they are. On the other hand, if you know that anything that you do is good, and you keep doing this, not only does everything go well, but also you begin to know what goodness truly is. Not only do you become that goodness, you are that goodness in life. So if you turn back to the good, it is because you make a decision and act in goodness for yourself.

"If you have trouble doing good things," the old people would say, "join a good group of people." In other words, join a group of people who are good. "If you join others who are good and who like to do good," Grandma Mary often said, "put aside your pride, follow their example. Only good can come of it. When you do this, you know that you can follow their teaching and their nurturing, because you know them to be good. When you walk with others correctly, life becomes swift, easy, and secure. That's because only high thoughts and high actions tend

91

to be done by good people. You must learn, however, to use your inner strength. Just remember that everything on earth here changes. For every good thing that you do, there's a chance to do something bad. It's important not to be confused by this, but to follow everything in action that leads to the good. Be honest and have courage."

So, I took Grandma's words to mean that if we really, truly do have difficulties in following that which is good, it is good to join a group of people whose thought and action always leads toward the good. Life becomes easier because you can be nurtured, taught, and protected by that.

Grandma would also point out that sometimes we can surround ourselves with people who are unstable, who constantly reverse themselves from doing good to bad things, from bad to good things. These people cannot control what they want. When they do something bad, they turn back because they resolve to do something better. But then again, they fall back to wanting something, desiring something. Grandma would say, "This isn't really all that bad, but it can cause great confusion and bewilderment. As long as you know that you can always return to that which is good by looking at your actions and by knowing yourself from what these actions have accomplished. You can always have a path back to that which is good."

Remembering Grandma's words, I find them to be true even when you encounter those times when things are truly, truly bad in the world around you—when people fool you because they want to, or people injure you because they want to, or people talk against you because they want to. It does not make sense to try to change them back to good. They have chosen the way of the bad people. In those times it is best to just hold to yourself. Do not show them that you are good nor boast about your goodness, just hold to your own center. And if you are in a group of people composed of the weak, the inferior, the bad, reconnect yourself with friends who know *Tunkasila,* who know *Wakan Tanka.* Knowing how to do this will make you turn back alone to the goodness. It is best that that decision be made by you alone, anyway.

Grandma was fond of saying, "When you return to that which is good, try to think nothing of being rewarded or being punished. Turning back to this goodness always brings its own reward. Be careful about the unexpected things confusing your mind, making you lose your sense of well-being, your sense of goodness. When you return back to the good, all you have to remember is to find the quiet space in your life. Learn how to keep still. Know how to come and go at the right times. Know how to rest. Know how to behave. Know all that light that is good in your life!" She said, "And the reward of this will keep unfolding!"

I took that as a lesson from Grandma about becoming calm even when I have to face the outside world. In doing that, I found that I do not see the struggle and turmoil of individuals. Instead I experience a true peace of mind that helps me to understand those great laws of the universe and of the sacred world. This understanding gives me the opportunity to act in harmony with others. I learned from Grandma that whoever acts from those deep, calm levels makes no mistakes. And if mistakes are made, they can be corrected.

So when the time presents itself to return to the good, it does not really help one to make excuses or to stay in the

93

triviality of things, but to truly look within and examine one-self in terms of those actions that one takes. If you do something wrong, you have to have the resolve to not only confess that wrong, but to have the determination to correct it. Taking that road removes you from regret and actually turns you back into a new way, a new direction that gives you a sense of a rebirth.

A rebirth only returns you back to the opportunity to do good things, to do loving things. And this kind of rebirth also requires you to take your caution to its fullest meaning. Just because you have returned to the good does not mean that it is an active part of your life yet. So you have to understand that what you have at the point of return are good intentions. Those good intentions are not strong enough to actually take shape and be understood in the world. You are still in the position where other people distort what you do, and they put their own ideals and thoughts to what you do. So the caution that you maintain allows you to go step by step in this correction. It is a position in which you should not try to force anything, but make certain of your relationships so that confidence is regained. Then, if you apply diligence, faith, and conscientious activity without attract-ing attention, your goodness begins to take root in the mind again, and obstructions to what you do fall away.

Grandma also used to tell me that we are given few oppor-tunities in life to return to the good, even though there are opportunities always available. We, by mistaken thought or action, can miss those opportunities. When we miss those kinds of opportunities, we experience bad things from within and from the world around us. If we find ourselves missing an oppor-tunity to return our lives back to the good, we set ourselves on a path that suffers defeat and failure. This kind of failure certainly has its inner causes, and it comes from the wrong attitude from the world or toward the world. All the bad things you experience then come from this wrong attitude because it attracts its own kind. What I learned here is that obstinacy, if it's blind, causes all kinds of bad effects, and the consequences of this attitude are very much like self-punishment; we constantly bring that which leads to failure. So, if we have the opportunity to return our lives back to goodness, we have to do so by nourishing that which is right.

A grandfather of mine by the name of Frank Picket Pen was a very powerful spiritual individual. He made some great accomplishments in his life and also made some great mistakes, but I learned a lot from him. I frequently went on the prairie to go look for the horses that we all kept in one pasture together. Although all the horses belonged to different individuals, they were kept as one herd by agreement. Grandpa Frank had a few horses in the herd. I was fond of riding one of his horses in particular. So, I used to go get his horse and ride it without asking him. He would always confront me about this. He would always tell me that I had to ask permission if I was to use other people's belongings and possessions so that goodness would prevail in those relationships. I would always get a lecture because I would continue to catch his horse and go riding it.

What he would say to me was, "You know if you really wanted to do good things and learn the proper way to ask someone to use his belongings, learn to do that which is right, learn to do that which is good. You ought to be careful what you say. Whatever comes out of your mouth has impact on the world

95

around you." So he said, "Be careful what comes out of your mouth. And likewise be careful what you put in your mouth—eating and drinking. Learn to calm your great urges and, if you ask me for my horse, I'll let you ride that horse anytime you want. I just want you to do it correctly." When I finally learned how to ask permission appropriately, we had a good relationship up to the end of his life.

6

It Is to the Great Spirit First That I Pray

Wakan Tanka	Great Spirit,
Tokaheya,	In the beginning,
Cewakiye lo.	I send my prayer (to).
Wakan Tanka	Great Spirit,
Tokaheya,	In the beginning,
Cewakiye lo.	I send my prayer (to).
Mitakuye ob,	With my relations,
Wanin wacin nan,	I want to live and,
Cewakiye lo.	I send my prayer (to).
Wakan Tanka	Great Spirit,
Tokaheya,	In the beginning,
Cewakiye lo.	I send my prayer (to).
Mitakuye ob,	With my relations,
Wanin wacin nan,	I want to live and,
Cewakiye lo.	I send my prayer (to).

There are slight variations to this song which is used to signify the truth that it is the creator to whom we always direct our prayers first. It is normally sung immediately after the making the pipe sacred song. Also, this version for our ceremony is different in word usage and melody from the popular version used in *Inipis* and *Lowanpis* (night ceremonies).

In 1967, when I returned to Rosebud after that school year, the lessons about humility from Grandma were very strong. I spent the first week home reconnecting with my friends and my relations, visiting relatives, and trying to determine what I would do for the rest of that summer. Grandma said, "We need to talk."

So I said, "About what?"

She asked me, "Do you remember you said that you wanted to do a *Hanbleceya* (a vision quest) when you were home last?"

I said, "Yes?"

She continued, "Remember? I told you that words you speak about the sacred should never be trivial, that you must carry out what you say?"

And I said, "Yes, I remember you said that."

She said, "Well, it's time for you to go visit Adam Bordeaux."

Adam was a long-time vice-president of the Rosebud Sioux Tribe. He was also known as a healer, an Eagle-Medicine Man. This I knew about Uncle Adam, and here my grandmother is saying that I should see him!

I asked her, "Why am I supposed to see him, Grandma?"

And she said, "Well, you said you wanted to do a *Hanbleceya*. I heard you, and now, you must complete what you said."

In trying to connect to what she was saying, I asked, "How am I going to do that?"

"I have gotten you a pipe." She pulled out a pipe and said, "Here, take this tobacco. Adam will show you how to use this. But before you go to him, you need some tobacco, *kinnikinick.*" She pulled some out, mixed them, and as she put tobacco in the pipe, she leaned forward, contemplating and saying a prayer. She capped off the tobacco in the bowl of the pipe with what she told me was *Tatanka Wigli* (the fat of a buffalo). Sternly, she said, "I want you to take this and walk up to Adam's home. I have told him you are coming."

I walked to Adam's home, which was about two miles from my home. I went and knocked on his door. Adam's wife came to the door and opened it. She saw me with the pipe and yelled, at what seemed to be the top of her lungs, "Adam, you have someone here to see you!"

Uncle Adam came to the door and said, "Oh, you've brought a pipe."

I said, "Yes, and I don't know what I'm supposed to be doing." And then I told him that Grandma had said that I should bring this pipe to him, and that I was given this pipe by Grandma because I had said that I wanted to do a *Hanbleceya.*

So Adam said, "Come here, come on in." We went into his home, sat down at a table, and he said, "Stand in front of me here." And so I stood in front of him, and he said, "Extend your pipe." So I extended my pipe. Then he said, "Now turn around." I turned around in a full circle. "Now," he said, "touch my hands," and he held out his hands, palms up. I touched his hand with the pipe, one hand with the bowl and the other with the stem. He pushed gently on the pipe and said, "Pull it back. Now do it again." And then, once more, he said, "Now do this again." So I touched his hands with the pipe and then pulled it back.

He said, "One more time." So as I extended the pipe and touched his palms, he clasped it, with the bowl and the stem in his hand. Then he said, "Before I take this, what did you say to your grandmother?"

I told him that when I was home during spring break, I had told her that I wanted to do a *Hanbleceya,* and that at first, she got angry with me because she thought I was being trivial. She thought that I was making a joke about a sacred matter. But I had told her I was serious, that I really wanted to experience what this was.

Adam looked at me and said, "It is good that you're considering doing the old ways in your life. The *Hanbleceya* is a very difficult thing to do, because it is a time when you must spend within yourself to speak to *Wakan Tanka*. Speaking to *Wakan Tanka* is not to look for something out there," he said, "*Wakan Tanka* is everything. In you, outside of you, everything that you hear, taste, touch, feel." And he pointed at my heart and said, "That's where *Wakan Tanka* is known. *Hanbleceya* . . . you should speak to some singers and learn some songs that you can sing while you're doing this. And we will do this by the end of June."

So, I asked, "What do I need to do?"

He said, "You need to have tobacco ties. You need to get a star blanket. And we'll do an *Inipi* before you go do this. You must feed all of those who help you, and you must give to the people who help you, show your appreciation."

And so I asked, "How many tobacco ties?"

And he said, "For me, you just do these green tobacco ties, seven of them. You'll need some flags, with tobacco, and do two hundred of each color of tobacco ties."

I asked, "Each color?"

And he said, "Yes. Black, red, yellow, white, that's what the flags should be. And two hundred of each of those colors is what we'll need."

And so I said, "I will tell Grandma."

He replied, "They can make tobacco ties with which to help you in your prayers."

So I said, "Okay."

He was firm in saying to me, "I will say to you that if you have any doubt that you don't want to do this, now is the time to back out. My taking the pipe from you is only my way of saying I will help you."

So, toward the end of June, I saw Adam one more time. He told me, "Four days before you do this, you stop all food, all water, and if there's rain, don't go out in it. Don't be touched by this water. Stay within your mind as much as you can and truly think about why you're doing this."

After all the tobacco ties were made, the food was prepared by my mother, grandmother, and Christina. On the day that I was to go sit on the hill to seek a vision, we drove to Adam's place along the river at the Grass Mountain Community.

When we arrived at Uncle Adam's home, we noticed an old man named Jack Williams was there. As I walked to the fire where he was standing, he began to tease me. He said, "Oh, you know you can die out there. You might not have a vision, and you might have to do this again." He said, "When I did this, I was really scared. Are you scared?"

I said, "No, I'm sort of wondering what's going to happen, but I'm not scared."

And he said, "Now's the time to back out. We'll eat and say *Hau* to the Spirits, and you can go home."

101

As Uncle Adam came out to where we were standing, he said, "Stop teasing the little guy. He might be doing it better than you did it!" I had to laugh. Adam turned to me and said, "Get your stuff ready." As I got my stuff ready, he said, "Now we'll go in here," pointing to the *Inipi*. So we all stripped down, grabbed some sage, and entered the lodge. Grandma, Mom, and other women sat outside. It was one of the first times I heard a whole series of songs in an *Inipi* ceremony, and Adam said, "The Spirits are waiting for you."

The weather was beginning to build up. It began to rain, not a thunderstorm but a steady drizzle. I was told to sit in the *Inipi* lodge so that the rain would not touch me until I went to the hill. As we finished the *Inipi* ceremony, I was instructed not to say a word once the ceremony was over, and that no one was to go in front of me. As I came out of the lodge, an eagle feather was tied to my hair. The star blanket was placed over my shoulders. I was completely nude, but I had to have my shoes on to walk to the spot that Adam chose, which was about three miles from his home, up on a ridge overlooking a river.

The other men who were there, three older men and some young men, all grabbed the tobacco ties and flags. As my father showed up, we started walking up the hill and Grandma came with us as far as she could. When she could not come any further, she just said, "Pray hard for me, for your relations, for those who went before you, and pray for your mother." She stopped at the top of the hill and watched us as we went on further up the ridge to my chosen special place.

Once at the site Uncle Adam picked for me, we stopped. Uncle Adam pointed at the place where I would spend my inner time. He marked out the spot with his feet. The flags were set in

the four directions; an altar was made of dirt on the north side
of the sacred spot that was being created. It was encircled by
tobacco ties. As I stepped in, they took my shoes.

As I stood there in my place, Uncle Adam said, "Son, what
you're doing is very sacred. Talk to *Wakan Tanka,* and *Wakan
Tanka* will talk to you. Ask *Tunkasila* for guidance to know the
person that you must know. You might experience some unusual
things. You might be endangered. You might get cold because it's
raining, and you might want to come back to the lodge." He
said, "There'll be a fire waiting, and these tobacco ties that are
around you are not chains. They are there to put the boundary
on the sacred place. To keep evil spirits outside of your sacred
space. To hold the sacred within. But they are not chains. If you
falter, if you do not want to continue this to its conclusion, just
break the south side of this circle in the white section. Break this
and walk back down. You will not be seen as a failure, but we'll
help you. We understand that you can only go as far as you can
go. But if you finish this," he said, "we will come after you. We
will talk to the Spirit, and you will tell the Spirit what you experienced while you were here."

I nodded my head. He said, "When we leave, do not look
upon us. Start with the West; pray to the *Wakinyan* (Thunder
People), and *Sunka Wakan Oyate* (the Horse People) who work
with them. Come to your center, go to the north. Pray to the
Tatanka Oyate (Buffalo People), who gave of themselves so our
people could have warmth, food, weapons, and homes. Look to
the east after you return to the center, go to the east. Ask the
Sinte Sapela Oyate (Black Tail Deer People) and the *Hehaka Oyate*
(Elk People) for guidance and help in all of your relationships.
Those people show us what is right and show us the temptations

of relations, so ask for their teaching so that you might know what is appropriate in those things. Look to the south, after you return to center, and ask *Wamakan Skan* (all that live upon this earth and within it, those who crawl in it, those who fly above it) for an understanding of all things. Come back to the center. Look above you and ask the *Wanbli Gleska* (Spotted Eagle) for vision, for clarity, for foresight, and for an understanding of the hidden strength that lies in all of us and in all things. And finally, look to your feet. Give honor and appreciation to *Unci Maka*, the mother who sustains you, who holds you, who helped to give you life, and who gives you all the opportunity to live this life each day. But," he said, "when you come back to your own being, begin to understand that *Wakan Tanka* is there. If you understand that *Wakan Tanka* is there, your prayer is heard. Call upon this life and His forces. Give thanks but vow to go forward. Anything that happens up here, just point your pipe, whether it be a living thing or a Spirit that comes to visit you. Keep them outside of your circle. This is your space. This is your time. And," he said, "we will come after you when we are ready." Then he laughed, "Of course, you'll see us if you decide to come back down! This is your prayer time." And he walked away.

I saw them walk down the hill. I was trying not to keep my eyes on them, because I was told not to. But I could see their figures in the enclosing darkness. After I saw that they were gone, I began my songs and my prayers.

The whole sum of my experience was one of hearing animals—coyotes, deer running by, and a dog walking by once. Then, as I got wetter and colder, and I could not sleep, the wind started up. Despite the wind, the west flag, the north flag, and the east flag hung limp, because they were wet. But the unusual aspect of this was that the south flag, the white one, was slapping my back. I was too petrified to turn around to see why it was blowing like it was blowing. The other flags were not blowing around at all! Toward morning, I realized that that is what I was to overcome, my fear of the sacred.

Without my glasses, I am not able to see anything clearly, but what I saw, I saw very clearly. I saw an eagle fly toward me, fly above me, turn, fly west, turn, come back, fly toward me. I had difficulty seeing clearly any shapes or forms around me, but I could see this eagle very clearly.

As the dawn was starting to show, I started to sing a song because I was gaining confidence, despite being cold and feeling that I should stop. As I started to sing this song, an aunt of mine who had passed away two months earlier came into my mind. And as I was singing, all of a sudden I heard her as I would hear a person standing next to me singing. That at first frightened me, but then I realized that this was one of those unusual things that I was to accept as a happening. So I kept singing the song. Her voice was loud, clear, and right there with the song I was singing. Her reputation as a singer was that she was loud. She was very strong in her singing. I heard her voice.

Daylight came, and after what seemed like hours of daylight, I heard voices. I was sitting in the middle of the circle because I was too cold and too weak to stand up. Besides, I did not want to be made colder by the winds. I had a wet blanket wrapped around me.

My dad, Uncle Adam, and Jack Williams walked up, and they did not say anything. They just broke the tobacco ties, wrapped them up, and pulled up the flags. They pulled the altar, destroyed it. Then, Uncle Adam said, "Walk in front of us. Don't

105

look back to where you've been. Just look forward, and we will go to the lodge."

My dad was crying quietly; I could hear him. He was the first to walk up to me and see me sitting, I'm sure, a poor, wet, soggy sight. But I felt strong inside. When my shoes were put on me, I started to walk back to the *Inipi*. When I got into the lodge, they took my blanket and my mother handed me a towel through the lodge door. I wiped myself despite shivering uncontrollably. The rest of the men, bare naked, crawled into the lodge.

The rocks were brought in and my uncle was saying, "You did well. I'm proud of you. Now, you tell the Spirit, and us, what you experienced." And so I recounted all the things I'd experienced, including the song with my aunt, and the eagle that kept coming back and forth. When Uncle Adam started to interpret for the Spirit, he said, "There's only one thing that the Spirit is telling you. You will see an Eagle-Man. I have spoken." Then we finished the closing songs. I came out of the lodge. Jack recounted my story to the gathering there. We ate, and I went home and slept for two days.

What did I learn? I experienced *Wakan Tanka* as the force of my life. It is truly in all things and is all things. I learned that it is to this life force, this being in all of us, that we must always reconnect with and pray to first. And I learned, also, that commitments are powerful when you keep them. That is the way that I connect myself to spirit in this song.

7

A Sacred People Are Coming to See You

Wakan Oyate wan	A Sacred People,
Waniyank' u welo!	Is coming to see you!
Wayanka yo!	Look!

This song is sung to prepare the officiant of the ceremony to perceive and accept the arrival of the Spirit People into the ceremony. The words in the song speak of a sacred people coming to see you, and the command seems to be, "Look." In Lakota, again, the idea of *Wakan Oyate* signifies two realities. One is certainly entities aside from ourselves that exist simultaneously, as we exist. The Lakota call this the Spirit World. Through a ceremony, we open the doorway where the Spirit makes its appearance, sometimes through entities that have a relationship with our world. The reverse is also true when we open the door to the Spirit World; we make our appearance in that world. So this song, and all other songs, too, are a process of relationship-making, connection, and opening of the two worlds to each other. So the words signify the connection that is made where the *Wakan Oyate* make an appearance in this world, and we as living, organic entities make our appearance in the Spirit World. So that doorway is open both ways.

What I learned about humility from my grandmother was that in honoring truth, in holding truth above all things, when you give your word to do something, in order for that word to find meaning in the order of life and in the Spirit, you, the person who has given that word, must carry that word to its conclusion. That word's conclusion is accomplished by activity and actions that give that word meaning in the organic world. So what it means is use your actions to finish what you said you would.

Uncle Charlie Kills Enemy, as he was teaching me songs, would emphasize that when you open the doorway to the sacred, you have to know that the *Wakan Oyate* (Sacred People) come to see you. You, in turn, as a *Wakan Wicasa* (Sacred Man), go to see them. In other words, it is to have a view or to have a thought that both worlds are open to each other, and we make an appearance both ways simultaneously. They, the *Wakan Oyate* (Spirit People), move into this world. We, the material world, show up, making an appearance in that world. In order for this to happen, we as human beings must have a knowledge of our own physical and spiritual beings so that we can center them in the truth of all things. And we must center ourselves in the truth of all things, the way they are exactly.

We must set a direction for ourselves, a goal, a point at which we want to be organically. My Uncle Charlie, in teaching me songs, supported by the songs I was being taught by Moses Big Crow and others, emphasized that a person with a direction begins to embody a lasting meaning in life, begins to understand how things work. So, that understanding of the direction must lead the individual to dedicate oneself to that truth. The totality of what one has experienced leads one to understand the meaning of one's life through that dedication. Every human being has a certain capacity, a certain capability, a certain personality, a nature that defines or gives direction in how the life that is being lived will unfold itself in this material world. This is a law of each individual, the nature of each individual.

In one of the discussions I had about the Sacred Pipe and spiritual matters with my Uncle Leo Chasing In Timber, he talked about the holy people that he used to sing for: Frank Picket Pen, Frank Arrow Side, White Lance, John Strike, and a few others. He would say that anyone who begins to know what lasts in this world and has a proper relationship to the Spirit World has to understand that they have to stand solidly and firmly in a direction they have chosen, to become one with oneself and with the Spirit World. So, a person who begins to understand life cannot be rigid in belief or behavior, nor can they be unmoving in their character. In this way, the person understands independence.

Uncle Leo never seemed to tire of telling me that these older people he grew up singing for and praying with always told him that the times that we live in change constantly. We have to learn to adapt to those changes, but the nature in the law that is expressed through your being, they used to tell him, if it determines all the actions that you take, it allows you to change with

109
ℒ♥

the times and their demands. So it gives a consistency and a meaning to life.

Uncle Leo looked at me and said, "We are given gifts by the Spirit World, and we are truly whole people. We're complete people." He said, "If we seek lastingness too quickly, we always leave ourselves open for bad things to happen. And that cannot benefit you because what can last can only be created slowly and through much thought."

I had an uncle named Floyd Black Spotted Horse, the older brother of Uncle Leo. He was a dancer and a handyman. He was active for the community in raising his family. He showed me something one day that stuck with me. I was watching him fix a car. A spring dropped from the motor outside of the car. I watched him pick the spring up. He saw me and showed it to me. Holding it up so that I could see it, he said, "Look at this, this has kind of lost its strength." He pulled on the spring, and it stretched way out. It became limp. It had no strength. Staring at the spring, he said, "There's a way to make this work again, to have it be strong," and he pulled the spring as far as he could stretch it, so it almost appeared like a wire. It did not look anything like a spring anymore. He took a large screwdriver. He began to wrap the wire around the screwdriver, so that the wire formed coils. After the wire with its coils was wrapped around the length of the screwdriver, he pulled the wire off. He set one end of the coiled wire on the ground so that the other end was up in the air. He started to push on it. Looking at it, he would push on it again and again. Then he took a hammer and hit the top end of the coiled wire a few times. He finally pulled it up and showed it to me. He said,

"Now it's got some strength." The wire had been compressed to where it was flexible, but it was taut. The coiled wire had become a spring again. It was strong and flexible as a spring should be.

He winked at me and said, "If you want to make something work again, you've got to take it all the way to where it doesn't work, and then you can help it back to where it works again." What I learned from that, and from many stories shared with me, is that if we act too quickly on something without understanding its nature and its capability, and we attempt too much with it, we succeed in nothing. We fail to accomplish what we set out to do. We do not help that which we are trying to accomplish nor finish the intended work. So in order to regain strength for anything, our purpose, or our direction, we have to first make certain that our effort and the tools that we use are equal to what we are going to use them for. Otherwise, we will make a mistake. In a way, we have to look at the good things that a tool or our own efforts can accomplish. We then have to understand that the resolve or determination we muster to move toward that which we want to accomplish does not become a problem so that we hurry what we do.

If we are to overcome evil, we have to learn how to unite our strength and our joy in a correct way; that we do not give in to what we see as the obstacle or the evil in the situation; that we do not get carried into a battle with what we understand as that which is bad or evil. We must focus on making a forward movement in the good with some energy. And in this way, we begin to accomplish appropriately and with patience that which has to be done.

In the experience I had with my Uncle Floyd, I saw that he was patient and careful in his actions to help the spring to regain its strength and flexibility. I took that situation and applied it in my life as a teaching. Often we end up in situations that are abnormal. Our goodness and our personalities can exceed a situation in its nature or in its demand. When this happens, we might put ourselves in a position to try something that is beyond our strength. We avoid this by understanding what things are demanded in a situation, what things have to be done to balance and put the situation into proper perspective. We can control our strength and avoid overactivity. We should not allow ourselves to make the mistake of overdoing something. Great caution and great attention to detail are required of a situation in order to use our proper energies. We should know that sometimes we are put into positions in which we are not fit to do the things that are needed to be done. If we are extremely cautious when that happens, we can even make it through those situations.

In much of my youth I encountered many people who, because of their problems with alcoholism or addiction, seemed to be at the mercy of their own passions, desires, hopes, and fears as they encountered their world. I saw these individuals as lacking a certain consistency, lacking a certain stability. And because they were in this inconsistent state of being, I always saw these individuals finding themselves in distress of one kind or another. I would see them being humiliated by situations they did not foresee, and especially by unexpected things. What I began to notice even more was that the world around them provided these experiences to them. The situations that I saw those people in frequently were evoked by their own actions, their own belief systems, and their own natures. Seeing their experiences taught me that when we give up our lives to our wants, desires, and passions, we exhaust our resources before we actually can put energy into accomplishing anything worthwhile. We begin to lean on things that do not have stability, do not have a foundation in proper relationship, and do not have the capacity for completion. We can put ourselves in a situation where our energy can die out very quickly, because we exhaust it. And then, it is at that critical moment that life presents its greatest tests.

Having had many discussions with Uncle Leo about the spiritual ways of our people, I began to understand how the ancients, elderly people, and even he looked at life. If we are going to go after something as a goal or something to accomplish, we have to sit down and understand what is the correct way to accomplish that task.

My Grandma Lena used to say, "If you're going to go out and hunt, you ought to know where what you're hunting normally finds itself or stays, or where it goes. If you go out into that prairie looking in a place where there's no animals to hunt, you can expend a lot of effort and energy without finding anything, even if you are persistent, because you go into a place that has nothing, no animals. Your search will not be worthwhile. So if you don't go after something in the right way, all your efforts will find nothing."

What I understood about that is, yes, we are given a mind, and we are given a body to experience and to know all conditions in the world that we live in. So, if we pursue game, we ought to know where the game is. We also need to know what we are hunting so we can know where that which we hunt tends to

113

abide. And it is important that we apply our will in a very strong and consistent way. In other words, it is necessary to be adaptable and, in that adaptability, learn to be persistent with our strength.

"If we do things correctly," my Grandma Lena would say, "the Spirit World helps us. And what we seek, we find, if we're looking in the right place."

It is important that we try to meet a situation in what that situation requires and meet it appropriately with our under-standing and with our action. Then what is needed by that situation should be accomplished.

Throughout my youth, I noticed that my people loved to gather together and have meetings, especially the elders. My grandfathers and grandmothers, in their meetings, expended much energy and effort to talk about how to help each other, how to help the weaker ones, and how to unite the people to do good things for each other.

There was a common theme in the Lakota way that I learned from my Grandfather Robert and my Grandma Mary that was very, very interesting. Grandpa Robert used to say, "When we do these traditional things, we do them because we've agreed to have a common purpose, a way for all the peo-ple to unite their efforts and their minds to doing this good thing. These traditions that we do are not laws, they are not requirements. If we hang on to a tradition simply for its own sake, without knowing what a situation requires, we lose flexi-bility and adaptability. We lose the understanding of what a sit-uation requires for it to be finished."

He said, "When we try to unite the people, we have to convince them that what we're trying to accomplish is right for the most people." And what this means is we have to unite the weak with the strong so that the common effort is applied equally by all who take part in trying to finish what we start.

"If we only keep up relationships with those whom we think are better than others, we create an unstable situation. So when we try to unite all people through our traditions, what we are trying to do is to finish that effort that through the unity of all people, benefit comes to all people. That's why we have many times that we eat together, and we feed everyone, weak or strong. If anything we do does not renew the life of our people, there's no praise in that, and there's no fault in that, but nothing happens. So when we try to unite people, what we are trying to finish is a situation that stabilizes the unity of our people."

He said, "It's good to know that as you're growing older because you'll encounter many people weak and strong, and you have to find ways to work with both kinds."

So, I took that to mean that the traditions we do are agreements that we have, to bring order to our lives, order to our activities. If the traditions themselves become the only ways of doing things to accomplish worthwhile purposes, we lose ourselves in the traditions. We lose our understanding, and we lose the strength and energy we need to put into situations that need balance.

More importantly, what I began to understand in what the old people were saying to me is that if we constantly move about quickly and are in a state of constant hurry without calming ourselves, we lose our energies, our strength, and our understanding to meet the needs of any situation. My grandma used to say, "In those times, you go to the holy people to regain some strength, to regain some knowledge on how to calm yourself, and how to follow their way so that even the Spirit World finds favor in your efforts, and things will go well. Working with people can be a very difficult thing, but if you do it correctly, with your understanding, following the ways of *Tunkasila* in walking this good road, then you can teach each other. You can help and protect each other, and the world and our traditions can then keep up with the times.

"It's very important," she used to say, "for you to know this. If you understand this, the sacred people come to see you. And you see the sacred people, because you go to see them."

I would sincerely contemplate this. It means that I should attempt things that I understand, that I can finish, and that will lead to new things, so I can always strive for a higher being, and strive to be a higher being. But if I act beyond my ability, because I have a great desire or passion, I put myself in a position to accomplish nothing. If I keep my word and I am committed to keeping my word, the task needed to finish the goal of my word has an easier chance of accomplishment. I have found that it holds true!

8

I Have Somehow Arrived

Miye	I,
Toki wahi ye.	Somehow have arrived.
Miye	I,
Toki wahi ye.	Somehow have arrived.
Wiohpeya tanhan,	From the west,
Wahi ye.	I have come.
Miye	I,
Toki wahi ye.	Somehow have arrived.
Miye	I,
Toki wahi ye.	Somehow have arrived.
Waziya tanhan,	From the north,
Wahi ye.	I have come.
Miye	I,
Toki wahi ye.	Somehow have arrived.

Miye	I,
Toki wahi ye.	Somehow have arrived.
Wioheyanpan tanhan,	From the east,
Wahi ye.	I have come.
Miye	I,
Toki wahi ye.	Somehow have arrived.
Miye	I,
Toki wahi ye.	Somehow have arrived.
Itokaga tanhan,	From the south,
Wahi ye.	I have come.
Miye	I,
Toki wahi ye.	Somehow have arrived.
Miye	I,
Toki wahi ye.	Somehow have arrived.
Tunkasila eca,	It is Grandfather,
Wahi ye.	I have come.
Miye	I,
Toki wahi ye.	Somehow have arrived.

The Lakota believe strongly that the Spirit World is always unfolding. *Tunkasila* and *Wakan Tanka* are viewed as omnipresent, therefore present even before the Spirits make themselves known to the holy man sitting at the altar. This song is often called a *Wicakicopi Olowan* (Spirit Calling Song), but I have also heard it referred to as a Four Directions Song. For our ceremony we are using this as a recognition song of the Spirit.

Because the Lakota view of the Spirit World is one of acceptance of that world as present, simultaneous to our world, it is an accepted view also that the Spirit World is growing and developing, right along with our material world. When the Spirit talks, or the Spirit makes its appearance as an entity aside from your own entity, that relationship, as I am told by the elders, must be an honest and truthful one in order for the goodness and its potential to prevail.

One of my grandfathers used to tell me that anything you do, whether it is a ceremony, a ritual, praying, "Don't depend on what you want to give to the Spirit World in terms of the material world, whether it's food, money, clothing, beautiful colors . . . What you must know is that the *Wakan Oyate,* the Sacred People, only want things that are truthful, honest, sincere, and simple." He said, "It's not what you want to give to the Spirit that makes this relationship what it is. A simple prayer from your heart can accomplish far more than all the gold you give to *Tunkasila.* In your mind, you have to really understand that what you say to the Spirit, and what you hear from the Spirit World, can only be understood and expressed through your faith, truthfulness, and simplicity. What is truly in your heart, what's expressed with simplicity and with truth, will accomplish far more in our world than any material thing you want to offer to the Spirit World."

119

After I had done the *Hanbleceya,* I went to a Wacipi, a dance celebration, in Parmalee, South Dakota. This small celebration was formerly held along the creek west of the town in a natural park. Every summer, the communities of Parmalee, Upper Cut Meat, and He Dog would get together and hold a dance celebration there. It was a celebration where people who are leaders in the community, those who are honored, had their giveaways and their feeding of the people. My uncles and father, as the Red Leaf Singers, often went to sing there. Because the

Red Leaf Singers hold much of the traditional warrior songs and the honoring songs, they would be invited to these dance celebrations to sing for people, to honor them, and to support them.

An uncle of mine named Raymond Hunts Horses used to sing with Red Leaf from time to time. I knew that he had worked with an altar. At this dance, when all my uncles and my father had gone to feed themselves, Raymond and I found each other sitting at the drum. I was curious about the message from my *Hanbleceya,* so I took this opportunity to talk to him about it. I told him, "I just finished a *Hanbleceya,* and I was told that I would see an Eagle-Man, and the Spirit said, 'I have spoken.'" And I asked him, "*Leksi* (Uncle), do you know what that means? I understood that you do these ceremonies."

He gazed upon me and he said, "When you have an experience like you did, and you're told what you are told, you are going to do this work. When the Spirit says you will see an Eagle-Man, two things will occur. You will see and experience the world through the eyes of an Eagle, and you will help people in the ways of the Eagle. You become an Eagle-Man." He said, "When I was young, the Spirit told me the same thing, and so I help people through the ways of the Eagle Ceremony. The color that the Eagle People want when you put up an altar is the color of the sky, blue-green, turquoise. These colors you must always use, and in your prayers, listen very closely to what the world is telling you. You will get your number from there."

I listened very closely, and I asked, "What does that mean to use your color?"

He said, "When people give you tobacco ties as an offering to the Spirit World for you to help them, the Spirit gives you a number and a color to work with. Maybe your asking me these things is your way of finding out what you need to do to hold yourself in proper connection. So, listen to the Spirit World! You'll get your number, but the color you work with is the color of the sky. And on that day that you're asked to set up an altar, you will know what color to use, and you will know what number to use."

At the time I was talking with him, he gave me numbers of tobacco ties that are used for different occasions, which I discounted because I was certain that I was not going to have an altar. I did not want an altar, and I was somewhat surprised that I was supposed to follow the ways of the Eagle in ceremony.

I grabbed Uncle Raymond's attention again. I asked him, "Does that mean I have to do this right away?"

He said, "Oh, you will do this when you're ready, but the Spirit World doesn't need elaboration of activity. The Spirit wants your truth, your sincerity, and the Eagle Ceremony is a very simple one. When you're ready, and the Spirit World wants to talk with you and they want you to talk with them, they will let you know, most likely through another holy person or through another Eagle-Man. It's very important to pay attention. It might take you years, or it might be tomorrow, but," he said, "the one thing you must know is that you must simplify your ways and learn to be sincere, be honest. And, into a ceremony, you should never take your anger and your animal feelings" (which I understood to be instinct) "especially, into any circle. Like the Eagle Spirit that you will work with, you must learn to rise above the world. You must learn to see far. You must learn to go after what you know. You must go after that which you know you must do.

121

"The first thing you must learn to do to be in the center, at the altar, is to know how to handle the anger that we develop when we relate to others. Bring it to stillness. Avoid acting in anger." He said, "It's very important that you also learn to lay aside your wants and your needs so that your life can regain its proper energies. So put anger to stillness and restrain your animal feelings so that your higher thinking, your connection to the Spirit World can open. This requires that you know how to complete that which you start without demanding much of others. When people ask you for your help, they know not to demand that which they cannot get, but they know that you can help them in certain ways. You have to learn how to be unselfish, learn how to be good. Learn to use your strength to serve others. It's best not to brag or make much of that which you're asked to do by the Spirit World. Learn to help quickly where help is needed, and truly and carefully, look at how much you can accept in terms of help yourself. When people help you they can harm themselves if they go beyond what they can help with. When you help others, make certain that you're helping correctly and appropriately. And develop good feelings, at the least, so you can give yourself without condition and without hesitation to the help that is most appropriate to be given. When you do this, you learn from the Spirit World and the wise ones how to put aside the mistakes that any beginnings and youth tend to make." He said, "You must look at your life experiences as teachings to do this correctly. It's very, very important that you listen to the old people in the world around you to know what is needed. So," he said, "allow yourself to be a young, foolish man. When you get beyond it, you'll learn when to sit in the center.

Learn to become a really good person and be thorough in that, and you'll do well. Learn how things work, learn the law."

Raymond, in telling me that I should know what is required in a situation and learn the law of the situation, also emphasized to me that no matter what we do, we have to get to a state of high-minded self-awareness and consistent seriousness if we want to be of service to others. We must make certain we do not forfeit any dignity. He thought that many people in the position of serving the sacred, or serving people who wanted something from the sacred, stood the danger of throwing themselves away in order to gain either position or validation for the service they were doing. He thought that it would be best if we maintained ourselves in our strengths, in our abilities, without diminishing our own space, our own position.

123

"And this is necessary," he said, "to be of benefit to others, especially if the benefit we are to give is to last. If we throw ourselves away, that is wrong! If we want to be of service, true service, and have lasting value to others, we must serve the Spirit. We must serve others without throwing ourselves away, without relinquishing ourselves." He thought that this was the best way that we could nourish what was right. That which is right, that which is correct, in turn nourishes us.

Uncle Raymond also said if we didn't nourish what is correct, we would lose what we were given and allowed to have by the Spirit World to do this service. If you were truly serving other people, you worked hard to provide your own means of nourishment. In the Lakota tradition, if you are serving other people you are supported in the proper way by the sacrifice of the individual who gives something to you for the service you are providing. They do this through the giveaway, or a feast for those who help. It becomes a duty for someone who asks for something of you to provide for you. Raymond said if you can't support yourself, you lose your ease, you lose your simplicity. Because in a way you shirk the proper way of making a living, and you begin to accept support from those who seek ceremony or ritual or from those in a higher position than you who want to use you for their own gains. He thought that was not a worthy way to make a living. It would make you deviate from your true self, your nature. And he thought that if this was kept up indefinitely, you would truly lose all the gifts you receive from the Spirit.

124

He also said that we must make certain that those whom we serve and those who serve us are entered into a relationship that is proper for all concerned. He said when many people gather together, jealousy and envy become real dangers. He thought that a proper relationship with those who ask you to serve them became a very close bond if the relationship was correct. And he said if you don't have those kinds of relationships, "Seek them out. Find those people who support and aid you and complement your work with their own service." And if you have relationships like this, he thought we could fend off criticism, envy, and jealousy. He truly thought that we could always learn something from the past, from the old people who knew how to work to get along with others.

When you begin to open the way in ceremony, and obstacles and hindrances are cleared away for yourself and for others, all the rules in that ceremony, in that service, begin to act in the same direction.

"It's like teamwork," he said, "and then the only danger you have to watch out for is weakness. It is important for you to maintain your stability, your firmness, your strengths, and your capabilities. Because without them," he said, "the danger of things falling apart is always a threat. And as you go forward in serving others in this way, learn some skills of how people are, how the Spirit World is, but in the skills you learn, keep those that will take you forward. And at all times, protect yourself against unforeseen attacks. You can do this by setting a direction, a path, a goal that you're striving toward that maintains harmony."

He said, "If jealousy prevails, everything tends to fall apart.

"In the process of getting to your own center, where you must be at the altar," he said, "you must constantly work at removing your faults, your weaknesses. It allows other people to come and share joy with you because they know you're working toward a position of no fault. If you have many faults, people who would otherwise be very helpful to all people through ceremony and ritual will stay away." And he said, "Sometimes the weaknesses you have, the faults that you have, get reinforced by the place in which you live or the environment in which you live." He said, "We must learn always to stay in humility because when we are humble we can see our faults, and we can give them up. And those who would stay away from you are relieved. Pressure is taken off of them and they approach with confidence. When they do this, there truly is mutuality in joy and in pleasure. So it's important," he said, "when people come approach you, even those with different views and even those who oppose you, you must learn to unite in good ways. When you don't have conflict with others, but you find viewpoints that separate you widely, great things cannot be undertaken or accomplished. Those points of view have a wide gulf between them. So when those who oppose you, but still need your help, approach you," he said, "you must understand that you should take things slowly, work yourself in small ways to produce that which can be accomplished, so that that which needs to be done is made more possible by what you accomplish. Those who oppose you don't necessarily mean that they're not in agreement. The need is created for agreement, so you learn to work toward it.

"Sometimes," he said, "when people oppose you openly, it's useful and it's important. So if you look at life, the Spirit World and the material world at the beginning oppose each other. Your spirit, your nature, finds itself in opposition to all Spirit and the nature of things." He said, "Look at man or woman, they're different in nature and they have to work out their differences to unite as one. When man and woman work this out, life is created, and life is reproduced. We live a good portion of our lives in opposition," he said, "this is just the nature of things, but these opposites in the world point out differences by which we can put things into their place, and that brings order into the world. So it's important to know the difference between opposition in viewpoint and conflict. Conflict is rarely, if ever, resolved. But people who oppose each other from divergent viewpoints," he said, "can get to a true, lasting, and significant harmony, a union.

"Sometimes the Spirit World and the world around you bring you something very good. If fate, if all the forces of your destiny, has marked a spot in time for you to get good," he said, "it comes without fail! This is not because you worked for it;

there are just points in life where the good comes from the highest places without your effort. When this happens, all you need to know is that you must put fear away because this kind of blessing comes from a place far beyond human weakness and human envy. When this happens, it's also very important that you maintain truth so you can keep uniting people, uniting their will, uniting their energies, so they can do great things together."

It is important to possess truth. Regarding this, Uncle Raymond was very soft in telling me, "You must work yourself to a position in life where you hold things together by the power of your character, the power of your personality. When your character is so strong that you can influence all who approach you appropriately, you will find yourself as you need to be. You can unite and hold together all those who think the same way you do, but you need this truth as a centering force in your life because anything outside of you that you can unite, without that central force of your character, begins to be deception, and it will break down at decisive moments in your life. So hold yourself together," he said, "make yourself strong in every way. Put your fear aside and when good things come to you as a blessing from the Spirit World, accept it. You may not even deserve it, but it's given without condition, without restraint, so it's important to know how to use this blessing in your relationships with others in correct ways."

He said, "In time, when you can sit at the altar and talk to the Eagle that you will see, and the Eagle who will see you, and the Eagle who will see the world through you," he said, "you'll learn how to bring benefit to the world without depriving others. When you know you can do this with consistency you

127

must learn to persist in this way, but even that requires a direction, a path, a road. If you become one of the people who gives out help and blessings to the whole world, this increase in energy that comes through you is intended to benefit the whole of life. This kind of blessing from the Spirit World does not take away from others, but you, sitting in this position, have to know how to persist in work consistently, with great persistence, to accomplish those things that need to be accomplished. And to find the help that you need. But what you accomplish with the correct help from Spirit People and from the people around you is not your gain alone. It is a good and a blessing that extends to all things. And this is available to everyone at all times," he said.

"That's why, when you sit at the altar, people can have confidence that the Spirit truly speaks through you, and you speak from the people to the Spirit World. But your real job when you begin to talk with the Eagle People is to make this blessing available to all. And in this way you'll know how to set boundaries, you'll know how to set limitations." He said, "Human perfection is not an ideal. Human perfection is all of our strengths and all of our weaknesses. But in order to work properly in relation to this perfection of life, we must know what we can be loyal to, and we must know what we must be disinterested in. Everything has a boundary, has a line, and these boundaries and these lines around things may appear troublesome at times, but they are effective in keeping a balance in life."

As I listened to Uncle Raymond, I remembered some of my Grandma Annie's words. "If you know how to save things," she said, "you're prepared for the times when there is lack, a want. If you know how to save things and how to spare things, it will save you from humiliation."

Uncle Raymond's voice comes back … "Look at the world again around you," he said, "the Spirit People, the Eagle People, realize that you will see through them, and they will see through you. One of the first things they will ask is that you have the appropriate boundaries for your life. And they will tell you to look at the world and its conditions. Look at the seasons. Every season has a fixed time. Day has a fixed time; night has a fixed time. And these fixed lines, these boundaries, give time in the year its meaning. Look at what you're able to gather together—for instance, money. If you let it flow through your hands like water and you don't save it to use properly, you'll find that it injures you. But if you know how to set a limit on what you receive and give out, for it to benefit you, it will preserve the things that you have, and it will save you from injury. So when the Spirit People and the Eagle People ask you to set your boundaries and set your limits, your lines that you put around yourself, even they must have balance. If you go around trying to impose strong lines and boundaries around your own nature, you will find you injure yourself. On the other hand, if you want to go out and go too far in requiring people to set their boundaries without allowing their growth appropriately, you will find that they will rebel against you. So," he said, "it's even necessary to have a balance with your own sense of boundary, your own sense of limit.

"So when you sit in the center, and the Eagle People begin to speak with you, always be ready to examine the nature of good. Especially help people do good and look at behavior, always that is correct." He said, "The only way that we can achieve significance in connection to the Spirit is to learn how to discriminate and set the proper boundary for the Spirit World in relation to you and you in relation to it. We have to know

129

what is good and what is evil. We have to know capability, ability, and how far we can stretch things, but we must also know how to define and discriminate the difference between good and evil. In the world, this is the backbone of people's behavior. The rules of conduct, the rules of behavior, morality. When you look out in the world, when you look at a tree, and you see its beauty, and you see its perfection as a living entity, when you wake up one day and realize that the beauty and perfection of that tree came about because of the boundaries that define what it is, you'll realize that life is not meant to be a path of unlimited possibilities. Unlimited possibilities for human kind would make human kind dissolve into the boundless. We have to know how things are defined by what has to be done in each situation, and we must know how to accept the boundaries of a situation simply because they are there. We attain free spirit when we surround ourselves with these boundaries, and by these boundaries, we determine for ourselves what our duty is in that situation."

He said, "This leads to the proper relationship between you and the Spirit World, between you and the service you provide, and it allows people to know what to ask of you because your conduct, your behavior, will show them."

I sat with Uncle Raymond a bit longer. I was filled with thought about what we had just discussed. I suddenly wanted to sing for the sheer pleasure of singing! If I am to talk with the Eagle, let it be another day! But I realized the impact of what Uncle Raymond had just said. The Spirit will just have to arrive when it wants to; I will talk when I am ready!

9

Everything Is Sacred. Look Here!

Kola!	Friend!
Canunpa ki le	This Pipe
Wakan yelo!	Is sacred!
Ehe k'un.	You said this.
Letunwan yo!	Look this way!
Kola!	Friend!
Canunpa ki le	This Pipe
Wakan yelo!	Is sacred!
Ehe k'un.	You said this.
Letunwan yo!	Look this way!
Kola!	Friend!
Lena ehe k'un!	You said these things!
Letunwan yo!	Look this way!
Kola!	Friend!
Wakaneja wan!	A child!

Ehe k'un.	You said this.
Letunwan yo!	Look this way!
Kola!	Friend!
Wakaneja wan!	A child!
Ehe k'un.	You said this.
Letunwan yo!	Look this way!
Lena ehe k'un!	You said these things!
Letunwan yo!	Look this way!
Kola!	Friend!
Wica Wakan wan!	A holy man!
Ehe k'un.	You said this.
Letunwan yo!	Look this way!
Kola!	Friend!
Wica Wakan wan!	A holy man!
Ehe k'un.	You said this.
Letunwan yo!	Look this way!
Kola!	Friend!
Lena ehe k'un!	You said these things!
Letunwan yo!	Look this way!
Kola!	Friend!
Lena	These
Wakan yelo!	Are sacred!
Ehe k'un.	You said this.
Letunwan yo!	Look this way!
Kola!	Friend!
Lena	These
Wakan yelo!	Are sacred!
Ehe k'un.	You said this.
Letunwan yo!	Look this way!

Kola!	Friend!
Lena ehe k'un!	You said these things!
Letunwan yo!	Look this way!

The Spirit World comes into mystical contact with our world by giving gifts of creativity and meaning. The Lakota believe one of the greatest gifts that the Spirit World can give to you is a gift of song. This song that we are singing now for our ceremony is the song given to me by the Spirit World. To keep a connection to the Spirit World, I am required to sing this song at every ritual or ceremony that I am requested to do.

At the time I started to do ceremony and ritual, I began to have inklings and direction from the Spirit World about the colors to use in ceremony and about the number that I was to use that would be significant when I set up an altar. The Spirit, in a ceremony, gave me the number 16. When a person asks me to do a ceremony, if they follow the forms and propriety in the Lakota tradition of asking for help in these ways, they bring the cloth, green-turquoise, six inches wide by three feet long, with sixteen tobacco ties of the same color tied to one of its corners. The person brings this, aside from the major cardinal colors and a number of tobacco ties to be used to encircle the altar at the ceremony. After we set up the *Owanka* and *Hocokan,* there is a time in that ceremony when these are used and I must acknowledge the gifts of Spirit to me personally, so I can in turn share them with those who ask me for help, or are praying with me within the context of the ceremony.

About four years after the altar was opened to me, I had a profound vision at the Fools Crow Sun Dance, in Kyle, South

133

Dakota. In broad daylight, I experienced what I now perceive as the voice of creation, the voice of *Tunkasila*. It challenged me to take a long walk.

The voice challenged me to put away all rational thought, all analyzing and reason I was using to try to understand, to comprehend my relationship with the Spirit World. And the same voice, in broad daylight, at the Fools Crow Sun Dance, told me to give my life to *Tunkasila*. It told me to give it as an expression of *Wakan Tanka,* and offer myself, offer to *Wakan Tanka* that which is truly my own to make a turning point in my life.

In 1985, instead of going to the Sun Dance, I had friends of mine from the Taos Pueblo strike down a cottonwood tree for me. We gathered many chokecherry branches. We tied them to the cottonwood tree. North of Questa, New Mexico, we put this tree up. I spent the day in prayer with my family and friends who came from many different places to support me. Without a singing group, but by offering my flesh, I pierced and prayed to *Tunkasila*. I offered to sacrifice my will and offered to *Wakan Tanka* my life. And in that prayer, the vision I had at Fools Crow Sun Dance was expanded.

As I stood, facing the north, a bee came buzzing by. It flew past me toward the center of the tree, flew back, hovered about six inches from my face and distinctly said, "Hello Howard! Why are you doing this?" The bee did not use my Lakota name, nor any of the names I use to be recognized by the Spirit World. It just called me, "Howard, what are you doing?"

Since the voice was so clear, I was thinking that one of my friends, who was sitting around the circle with me, praying with me, supporting me, had voiced my name to get my attention.

134

So, I looked around while I was pulling on the rope that tied me to the tree. The bee hovered there for a moment. When I saw it, it buzzed over my shoulder and disappeared.

I began to think in rational Western terms of what the bee stood for, what it symbolized. I was trying to find a connection to why this happened. As I was struggling with my need to understand this, a calmness, a quiet, came over my whole being. I heard a song! As I was hearing it, I realized that I had to pay attention, so I began to sing with it. I realized that this was a song that I was supposed to receive to unify my being with the Spirit World. This song, I was instructed, was to be used in every ceremony that I was conducting to benefit others.

This song makes the *Canunpa* sacred, but I must perceive it this way. Since the Spirits spoke in this way, I am to take this song as the Spirits saying, "This *Canunpa* is sacred. It is a way to walk, a way to be, but it must be seen from the center of one's being (my being)."

The Spirits said, "The children are sacred!" The song reaffirms, "Look here!" This is attributed directly to children who have yet to understand the difference between good and evil in the truth of all things.

The song says, "Holy people are sacred." And in the same phrase, the song says, "There is a way to be sacred. Look here." In other words, make an appearance here. See from the center.

The song finally tells us, "Everything is sacred!" if we see it from here in the center. And I realized that this song was recognizing my need to serve. I must be able to understand, and be able to rule that which is good in my own life. But to do this, I had to expect the Spirit to help. In that, I had to realize that the

135

Spirit, alone, truly has the power to help the world. It gives opportunity. It has no interest in controlling the world. Its greatest interest is to give opportunity to the world so that the world itself by its own will and choosing chooses the path of goodness, lastingness, and love.

In the Sun Dance, a man or a woman sacrifices from a high place, from a high thought, for the benefit of all those who want to live. And this sacrifice gives a sense of joy and thankfulness that is so necessary for the flowering of the people. When the people, through seeing this sacrifice, can follow the good, have a love of the good, and can unite with others to do great things, the most difficult and dangerous undertakings can be accomplished. Those efforts can be unified and goals can be accomplished with benefit to all.

What you learn of sacrifice in this manner, for the benefit of all people, is that the energy you get, the blessing that you get, and the help that you receive, finds itself in a limited time on the face of the earth. When you call upon it and it arrives, it becomes necessary through your service to work and to make best use of that time, because this time is a blessing from the highest of Spirit. This blessing, this energy that you are given unites the Spirit and material worlds, where the material world takes the creative energy given by the Spirit World and helps it to form and bring forth living and dynamic conditions and beings. In my own sacrifice, I learned that benefit given in this way does not endure. We have to use it quickly, while it lasts on the face of the earth. This lesson is for human beings to understand that when spiritual energy is called upon and brought into the material, unless it finds form, unless it finds manifestation and is utilized in this manner, that energy dissipates in time and goes back to where it came from. And to make the best use of this energy, I also found, is an opportunity to widen the view of the truth so that the world and its strengths, its weaknesses, its good, its evil, and its faults, can be accepted. When you understand this, you realize you have to use this energy, first to benefit yourself, in the sense of spiritual awakening, so you can share it with others. But as you bring this awakening into the world, you have to look at the world to discover the good in it as it shows up in others. In your own being, when you see this good in others, you learn to imitate it in order to make it your own. But if you look in that world and you see something bad, you perceive it so clearly because it also exists in you. You find that you have to rid yourself of it. You have to work to rid yourself of evil.

The greatest benefit to your character, to your personality, to your being, is this ethical change that frees you of evil. As you begin to serve the world, you have this view to serve the world in the best way that you can. The Spirit World, that which is high, begins to help you because you are making the correct sacrifice. This gives you an increase of strength to be used to achieve something that is not only beneficial but is great, and can last for a time. And because this energy is experienced, you have to make yourself ready to take the responsibility of seeing its manifestation in life itself. It is at this point that you learn to put your ego, your selfishness, aside. If you make yourself selfless, you bring about the greatest opportunity for yourself and others that is bound to produce good. It also puts you above blame; it puts you above fault.

As you contemplate using this energy, you have to understand the gift of the divine that shows up in the workings of the

137

universe. When you call upon this energy, this force in turn calls upon you to influence others in such a way that this goodness is produced in like effects, similar effects. You find that you have to contemplate, not only in a religious, but also in a spiritual manner, that which amplifies and strengthens your faith, because in faith, you know the mystery and the divinity of the laws of life. And by exercising the greatest inner concentration, you can give expression to these laws in your own being. It is true that when you begin to do this, others begin to sense a hidden spiritual power that emanates from you. They sense its influence and they feel dominated by you without their being aware of how it happens. So if you begin to serve humanity and all life with the call upon this force of life, this energy, you have to put yourself in the position where you have a view of the real sentiments of the mass of people around you, so that you are not deceived by them. But your being, through your action, must be so connected to those laws in their expression, that your being, with the impact of your wisdom, can influence those who are willing to be influenced in this way. They too can give themselves in service to Spirit and to themselves.

We must have the greatest outlook on humanity, without judgment, to achieve this kind of position. It is important that we give up everything that is related to desire. We cannot go after this energy with an intention because if we do, what we are showing the Spirit World is that we are only thinking about this from a distance, without understanding. And if our influence is not appropriate, then it certainly is not understood by the people around us. If we truly have brought this blessing into the world, the world around us doesn't have to understand this. This is true because our actions and our connection with the Spirit World helps those people whether they understand it or not.

But for ourselves, the Spirit World says that we should not ever be content with a shallow, thoughtless view of the prevailing forces. We must understand and know them as a connected whole. In this understanding, we must begin to influence our world toward that state of goodness and love.

What the Spirit has taught me through this song is that every person who has a real benefit in life gets this blessing from the Spirit World. If an individual produces in himself the conditions for this blessing, the Spirit World gives the blessing. The condition for this blessing is for one to have receptivity to, and a love, a genuine love, of the good. So when one strives for goodness, not for gain, fame, nor position in life, but only strives for goodness itself, that which one strives for comes of itself. This is the inevitability of natural law. When a blessing is given by the Spirit World to us, and we know it, we are in harmony with the highest laws of the universe and nothing, not even an accident, can prevent the blessing.

But the Spirit also tells me through the song that we have to be cautious and heed what this blessing requires. First, we have to make this blessing our own through inner strength and a commitment to persist in this goodness. If we accomplish this, we acquire meaning before spirit, creation, and the world. It only shows us that we can accomplish something truly for the good of the world. We can only do this because we learn how to forgive the world of its weaknesses. We learn to forgive our relations for their weaknesses. We learn to seek a correct relationship which has commitment, a correct relationship that is so firm it

139

can triumph over everything. We have to know how to forgive in a sense of allowing others to do their own good.

When a bird, a water bird, calls from a distance, the water bird's young answer it. It can be a long distance, but when this call is heard by the young ones they answer and they return back to the mother.

When you as a person in the service of others find that you have an influence upon persons of the same spirit, it appears involuntary. Though this appears as though it was not put forth as a calling, it is a calling. So, persons who share the same spirit hear the note of the message; they recognize it, and they answer by uniting with it. If you awaken an echo in others through spiritual attraction, whenever you voice with truth and frankness, and whenever you do something that is a clear expression of your truth and intention, the Spirit World says that a mysterious and far-reaching influence extends from you. So, it acts naturally on those who are receptive to it. As more become receptive to it, the circle grows larger and larger. So, the Spirit World, through this song that it gave to me, says that the root of all influence in one's own being comes from this connection to others through spiritual attraction.

If we give our inner being true and energetic expression through our words and actions, the effect of it is great because it reflects the very thing that our hearts have accepted and owned. But also in the song, the Spirit World says that any deliberate intention to produce that effect can only destroy the possibility of its manifestation. Grandpa Charlie Black Bear used to say, "Speak your words carefully and well. Many people will hear you. If you sit and you don't speak well, people far away will contradict what you say. What you speak goes from you and exerts influence on others. What you do begins from you and becomes visible far, far away. So what you say and what you do determine whether you are a holy being, a connected being. So," he said, "be careful what you say, be careful what you do. They will either bring you honor, or they will bring you disgrace. Just be careful."

When we receive a blessing and help from the Spirit through our service and our acceptance of the power of spirit to help the world, even what are considered bad events or unfortunate times turn to our advantage if we are affected by them because this blessing is so strong. This help from the Spirit, which is what is meant by a blessing, is so strong and so unobstructed that even bad things we experience while we're being blessed by the Spirit help us to become free of mistake, to become free of blame. But it is only by acting in harmony with truth that we gain such a position of influence that the Spirit itself does not contradict our intent. Of course, all this means is that we have to learn to walk our talk, to know what works, to put energy into our words by our actions, and our words should always be related to real things in life; otherwise, they become deception. This is what my Grandpa Charlie used to say, "If your words and your actions are like one, you can move anything, including the Spirit World."

We must understand that this blessing, this service from the Spirit to us, and our service to the Spirit in turn, only gives us the opportunity to treat our relations with the understanding of what works. In relationships, it is best to allow people complete freedom of movement so that we can minimize mistakes.

141

The blessing from the universe, from the Spirit, only allows us to create proper relationships.

One of the ways in which we know that we are using the energy for proper relationships correctly is how we relate within the family. In the family, we have the greatest opportunity to walk our talk, to make our words real by the actions that we accomplish.

In a family relationship, it is important to have a balance between being severe and being indulgent. If we are too severe toward our own, we can make great mistakes. If we know how to allow complete freedom of movement, of motion, for every individual in our family, but know how to keep order and balance, it leads to a great discipline. This does not mean severity; it means to use strength in our action appropriately because too great weakness in a relationship that needs firmness can lead to disgraceful situations. This, I was taught by my Aunt Christina.

On one of my visits home from school, my cousins LaVern and Ambrose, myself, and a few others got together and hopped in one car. We told Christina that we were going to go out partying. Among the Lakota, growing up in the times that I did, partying meant that you crossed the state line of South Dakota into Nebraska, to some of the small ranching towns to go buy alcohol. To party in those times was to get as drunk as you could. Numb yourself so you could feel a sense of power, feel a sense of influence.

Christina warned us, "If you're too rambunctious, too wild, don't come back here. Finish your party, then come back."

I think we heard her words, but somewhere in the middle of the night, we drove back to Uncle Leo and Christina's

142

home. In the midst of our having a great time, someone said something that upset everyone. As we pulled up to Uncle Leo and Christina's home, we all jumped out of the car and proceeded to have a big fistfight. Uncle Leo came walking out of his home. I could tell he was angry with us. He said, "All of you are acting like a bunch of pack dogs, and if you don't stop your fighting right now, I'm driving into Rosebud. I'll bring the agency police back here, and all of you will spend a day or two at the jail." And he was ready to go.

All of us left the car running and took off in different directions—off into the canyons. That was a favorite thing we used to do if we were caught doing something and we wanted to get away for awhile. We would run away into the canyons. I took off west of Uncle Leo's house into the canyon and passed out. The next morning, I came walking back to Uncle Leo's. Christina met me at the door. She let me in and she poured me a cup of coffee. Ambrose was already there. LaVern was still nowhere to be seen. She said to me that when we were drunk like this, we were difficult to restrain.

She said, "It's better if you learn how to discipline yourself, so external restraint isn't applied to you." She said, "That causes disgrace." I took that to heart.

If we honor order within our own being, we honor order in our relations with others, especially our close relationships, and that leads to greater honor. In the process of utilizing the blessing and help from the Spirit, there are times when we are put in a position to mediate the disagreements and arguments that others, leaders and followers, young and old people, get into. If we have this blessing from the Spirit, we learn to have

143

disinterest in the positions taken by those parties and individuals, since the benefit of the blessing that we are to spread to them must be an understanding of that which creates order and renews life. If we are to mediate between disagreeing factions, we learn to give this benefit from the Spirit in a selfless way; everyone should benefit, and this blessing should really reach those for whom it is intended.

If we act as this kind of intermediary in any situation in life, we must be willing to own our influence on others as a sacred event because if we help disagreeing parties come to agreement, it helps them to accomplish great things. They become decisive for the future, and the requirement for their agreement is assured. This is only done by reducing fault in the situation in all parties involved, whether they are influential or not. Reducing fault in the situation requires purification, a return to goodness, a return to understanding how to unite individuals and their minds into a common agreement.

My Grandpa Frank Picket Pen used to say that in Spirit and in the material world, we cannot ever lose what really belongs to us even when we throw it away. It is important not to be anxious about what we own, especially those things that abide within us. When there are disagreeing factions, we must let them know this truth; that in coming to agreement, they should learn to remain true to their own nature, not listen to the falsehood of others, and be able to come to agreement so that this agreement leads to the accomplishment of great and lasting things.

In the blessing and benefit from *Tunkasila,* a certain reality has to exist in how we use this blessing. The old people tell me that in truth we must strive for kindness at all times. Kindness

144

always has the effect of recognition, and benefit, and blessing to all who are influenced by it, because true kindness does not count upon nor request merit and appreciation. True kindness only acts from necessity. Among humans, it acts from inner necessity. Kindness is always rewarded with kindness. And kindness, like all human endeavor, has to be nurtured, not for reward, not for merit, but simply for its own sake.

Over time, I began to understand my Grandma Mary when she would say, "Be careful, and humble yourself." I realized that in beginning to understand ourselves, the person we have to learn to love before we learn to love any other is ourself. In that love of self, we must exercise kindness to ourself. If we accomplish this, this is what we give in turn to the world around us. In coming to being kind to ourself, we might be conscious of a lack or deficiency in the self, especially when we know that we have to nourish all people through a task given to us, like serving the people in the altar. When we recognize a lack or deficiency in ourself, we realize, initially, that we cannot nourish the people because we do not have the strength to do it. It is at those times that as we free ourselves of ego, we sit down and beg counsel and help from anyone who is spiritually superior to us. We seek not from one who is higher in elevation, but from one who is actually walking the path of spirit. We do this to return ourself back to the path of Spirit. If we humble ourself and remain kind to ourself, this attitude of mind and the persistence in it leads back to uniting thought and action in a correct and beneficial way. But at the time we are asking for help, we have to remain aware of our dependence. We need this help and so we have asked for it.

145

When we are being helped, it does not make sense to put ourself forward or attempt great things until we truly learn how to be kind and loving of ourself. On the other hand, if we return to that state, humility requires that we accept this and return to serve all of life. This I understand to be true.

When we abuse the blessing from *Tunkasila,* and when we manipulate this blessing and use it inappropriately, the truth we encounter is that we bring increase or benefit to no one. And we open up ourself to aggression and attack. And this becomes so because we do not keep our hearts steady.

If we achieve a high spiritual position in life, we have to renounce the material things of the world to bring benefit to those who seek our help. If we neglect this duty and help no one, we lose the furthering influence of others and find ourselves alone very quickly. So the world, in seeing our weaknesses, invites itself to attack us. If we have removed ourselves from harmony with the duty or the demand of the time, of a necessity, bad things will come.

The Spirit, through the song that it gave to me, says that we must perceive these truths as one truth and learn how to make the appropriate relationship, the correct relationship, with others and especially with the Spirit. Before we act, we should set ourself at a state of rest and calmness. If we want to speak, we should calm our minds, compose their rest. Before we ask for something, we should firm up our relations, whether it be with the world around us or with the Spirit. It is only by doing these three things that we gain a sense of security that is genuine. But if we are in a hurry and we are short with others in our actions, we find that no one will cooperate with us.

If we are angry and our agitation shows through our words, there is no echo in others. If we demand something or ask for something without having established relations, that which we ask for will not be given to us. Harm and injury come nearer when no one is there to support us, and, usually, that is of our own doing.

So, in situations where we have a rebirth, a turning point back to a state of goodness again, the elders always say, "Be cautious. Be careful. Humble yourself. Learn to value truth. Learn to love goodness." If we fail at this, or we give up our efforts to arrive at a state of goodness, we throw up our hands and arms in failure and defeat. We stop all effort to get to this point of harmony and acceptance of that which is good and that which is loving. What have we done? We are saying that the difficulties are too great. We are saying that we are stuck, that we cannot find our way out. So we are throwing up our hands, and we give up the struggle. All we are saying is "We have failed." We have resigned ourselves to be sad, to be weak.

All that the old people have ever told me about this mistake is, "Don't stay in this condition. Do not persist with this. Come back to yourself, be kind to yourself. Be humble, but be careful." This was truly an important lesson. When Spirit gave me the song, that is what I was reminded of: "Friend, remember you said these things. Perceive these things; let them make an appearance. Let it be so."

147

10

The One I Am Singing for Is Now Coming

Tuwa,	Who,
Waki lowan k'un?	(Remember) one I am singing for?
Wana u welo!	(He) is coming now!
Tuwa,	Who,
Waki lowan k'un?	(Remember) one I am singing for?
Wana u welo!	(He) is coming now!
Wana u welo!	(He) is coming now!
Wanka tanhan,	From on high,
Tunkasila,	Grandfather,
Waki lowan k'un?	(Remember) one I am singing for?
Wana u welo!	(He) is coming now!
Wana u welo!	(He) is coming now!

This song further amplifies the reality of the Grandfathers' presence. The Spiritual Leader at the center is about to acknowledge the arrival of the Spirit People.

Singing is the active part of making music with one's own physical body. How this connects to the sacred is that music made by the body generates an enthusiasm. It generates harmony; it generates confidence, so these things allow the will to be done in great things as long as there is a devotion to movement and activity with proper direction. The Lakota say that the Spirit World and the material world move in relation to each other, like in music. What is sacred, when it is moved by devotion, shows the people the easiest manner in which to get to correction.

The old people say, when they sing their song, that it is the most powerful way to unite the sacred and the material. They have believed that all natural and human law is activity and movement that meets with devotion. Those who came before us are united with us in ceremony through song. The ancestors with the truth of their beliefs, the present, and all who share the present, are united through rhythm and through the path that shows the least resistance. The future is brought into the present as a possibility, an opportunity, with devotion that will maintain confidence, maintain harmony, maintain a path with the least amount of obstruction. So, when the song says, "Who I am singing for now is coming . . . ," it is akin to saying that the centering needed for all things, past, present, and future, is beginning to arrive in its opportunity and possibility.

For those who seek answers outside of themselves, the words in the music would show the arrival of a force that will take care of things. For those who understand the rising, the appearance, and the coming from within, the greatest spirit that abides within, a song like this shows that these forces are now becoming evident. For one who looks to the future to know oneself, to have the confidence and enthusiasm to accomplish great things, this music says, "This can be." But music, in its harmony and the devotion of motion and activity that it generates, truly shows a rhythm, a happening, that can be directed to the accomplishment of great purpose.

The holy people, when they sit in the center, and know that the Spirit World and the material world are uniting, understand that a relationship is created where a doorway between that world and this material world is open. So we go into that Spirit World, and the Spirit in turn comes into this world, in a simultaneous movement. What this simultaneous movement begins to show is the activity and the movement of all beings that contain the harmony imminent in them, in proper relationship. Music releases tension and stress; it allows one to experience joy and to relieve the pressures of life. It allows emotions a free rein to lose their charge. So Lakota people look at music as truly serious and holy, in that music can be designed to purify the beliefs and feelings of all.

The Lakota rarely look at the failings and weaknesses of human endeavor in music. Through music, the greatness of the past is recalled. The opportunity for accomplishment, victory, is called upon in the present through song. The future, and its possibility for great accomplishment to be present, is willed through music. So, when the Spirit People, and those in the material world who sing for the Spirit World and the material world to come together, who you are singing for now, comes into the present.

151

This is the teaching of most of the songmen who have taught me sacred music.

It is a genuine acceptance of *Tunkasila* as present in all ways and in all things, past, present, and future. And since the true spiritual view is not to look at this *Tunkasila* and *Wakan Tanka* as outside oneself, all that *Tunkasila* and *Wakan Tanka* represent, along with *Unci Maka,* begins to appear in the moment, through song. Greatness is made possible by the sudden movement, with devotion, to follow a road that is least obstructive. It generates the activity, and it generates the possibility for all things to unite in the present in the most appropriate way with the least amount of obstruction. So, when I call upon *Tunkasila,* from on high, by singing for *Tunkasila, Tunkasila* comes into the now. Thus, in the ceremony, we (you and I) begin to experience the possibility and generation of enthusiasm to accomplish great things.

11

Their Voices
Can Be Heard

Hotainpe!	Their voices are clear!
Hotainpe!	Their voices are clear!
Wanka tanhan,	From above,
Hotainpe!	Their voices are clear!
Hotainpe!	Their voices are clear!
Wanka tanhan,	From above,
Hotainpe!	Their voices are clear!
Hotainpe lo!	Their voices are clear!
Wanka tanhan,	From above,
Inyanwan,	A Stone,
Hotainye!	Its voice is clear!
Hotainye!	Its voice is clear!
Wanka tanhan,	From above,
Hotainye!	Its voice is clear!
Hotainpe lo!	Their voices are clear!

As the Spirit People begin to make their presence felt and known, this song is sung. The word *tain* can be translated as "clear" or "heard." While the song is being sung, certain phenomena such as little lights, or blue flashes of light in the darkness can be observed. This then signifies to the holy man that other songs can now be sung so that the Spirit can be communicated with clearly.

At the time I had the vision at Fools Crow Sun Dance in Kyle, South Dakota, my Uncle Jim Dubray wanted my help on one of the evenings during the dance. We had finished for the day. His daughters and several other ladies had gone into an *Inipi* lodge to do their cleansing prayers. In the middle of the songs, one of Uncle Jim's daughters was entered by a Spirit, and she began talking in tongues. She was having a difficult time with the experience that was occurring in that *Inipi*. So, he sent someone to get me from my camp. I went immediately to stand by his side.

Upon my arrival, Uncle Jim said, "Son, I have a favor to ask of you, and I want your help."

And I said, "I'll see if I can help. What do you need?"

Uncle Jim walked in front of me to the *Inipi* where his daughters and the others were having their ceremony. Along the way, he told me that there was dissension in the camp between a few individuals, that one of the individuals had brought a gun in his car to the Sun Dance even though he was one of the leaders. The disagreement about this gun on the dance grounds led to a great dissension. Uncle Jim felt that all this dissension was affecting certain ceremonies that were being conducted throughout the evening. Now that he had seen his daughter responding to a spiritual event in this way, he thought that we should do something to address the situation.

We walked to the doorway of the lodge. Uncle Jim turned to me and said, "Son! Sing a song, a Four Directions Song, so we can ask the Spirit for help." So I stepped forward. I sang a *Tatioye Topa Olowan* (Four Directions Song) addressing the west with the Thunder Beings, the north with the Buffalo Beings, the east with the Elk and the Black-tail Deer People, and the south with all that moves on the face of the earth, the living things, the plant world, and all who walk, swim, and fly. We addressed all of them. Then we addressed *Tunkasila* above and asked the *Wanbli Gleska* (Spotted Eagle) to give us vision and foresight to help with the situation. We asked *Unci Maka* to hold us, to bear with the good things and the evil things that we were being confronted with. We further asked to have an understanding to use the proper energies to deal with this dissension, in this spiritual emergency that was occurring. The song I sang also said, "The people have fear, so help me that I may deal with this." I finished the song, and I stepped back.

Uncle Jim's sons, Tom and Steve, and a couple of other young individuals came and circled the lodge where this prayer was going on. Uncle Jim stepped forward. He shouted to the four directions and sang, "We need your help. We need it to bring calmness to this dissension and calmness to this fear that the people are experiencing." He raised his arm high. "Help me! Let me know what to do!" From the four directions around camp, the coyotes gave out two yells. I immediately had the sense that the Universe around us was responding to us.

It did not seem mystical, but certainly was an appropriate response to his plea. We prayed with firm determination. The next day, the individual who had brought the gun left camp. We began to experience a greater responsibility to bring harmony back to the dance.

During the dance the next day, my Uncle Jim said to me, "You must tie your *Cekpa* (umbilical cord) because *Tunkasila* will talk to you." Up to this time in my life, I had always been told that the Sun Dance was a vow that you undertook for yourself, for your people, and for whomever you were praying. You offered your life so that that person or your people, or what you were praying for was helped and resolved. I had this belief that no one could tell you to do this. Though I still have the belief currently, to this day, the challenge of that day was that my Uncle Jim had asked me to do this. I rebelled.

I encountered my greatest adversity as an inner oppression, an inner state of great difficulty and challenge. I am certain that this rebellion and inner oppression I was experiencing led to the vision that I had. The combined circumstances of that Sun Dance and the vision brought me to New Mexico, to offer myself, my body, to spirit. But in my rebellion, I guess Uncle Jim also learned that when *Tunkasila* asks you to do something expressed through a holy person, you have the right to say yes or no, but you must deal with what transpires as actual events to face and to resolve.

From that time, I began to understand what adversity and what difficulty in life mean. I understand now that they are opportunities to deal with the side of life where nothing is achievable, where difficulty prevails. Problems and troubles come in abundance. You can do nothing except to face them, regain your own strength, learn to be honest with yourself, and prepare yourself to truly talk with *Tunkasila* within.

The year after that event, I went back to Rosebud, South Dakota, to reconnect with my own people, the Brule, Sicangu. I went to the Hollow Horn Bear Sun Dance to make this reconnection. I offered my body to the Spirit. My vow was to pierce in the first piercing round of the Sun Dance, and to stay pierced and connected to the sacred tree for four days. I had planned to stay in the dance ground and to break my *Cekpa* on the last breaking round of the dance on the fourth day. That was the intention that I had.

Upon my arrival at the Hollow Horn Bear Sun Dance to offer this sacrifice, my uncle Albert White Hat and my cousin Duane Hollow Horn Bear offered the pipe to me to help them spiritually with the dance. I took the pipe. I vowed that I would help them and the people. But I needed to finish my sacrifice. I needed to finish my vow for the purposes of reconnecting with my own people since I had been away for so long. I had been working with the Oglala People in Pine Ridge for about seven years with their Sun Dance.

I pierced my body in that first round. I took a position on the east side of the dance ground with my rope, along with my sacred objects, attached to the sacred tree. The first day was difficult. During the first night I slept under the sacred tree that we are connected to during the Sun Dance. I had a buffalo robe underneath me. I had two Pendleton blankets and a space blanket, which was metallic and orange in color, to cover me. I wrapped myself tightly, but comfortably. I lay on my back, because if I moved, the pegs that were skewered through my chest would push against my body and it would hurt. So I took a position directly underneath the east side of the tree and went to sleep.

The moon was fully bright that night. As I was falling asleep, I began to have a long night of ancient elders and ancient people walking by the tree and touching it. In my mind, it was a dream. It seemed very real because faces I remembered in some of the people who came by would greet me. A number of the old people would stop and they would laugh. They would talk amongst themselves. They would point at me and whisper, "What is he doing? What is he thinking he's doing?" A couple of the old ladies who stopped at the tree looked over me. Standing above me, they said, "He's trying to sleep. But look at the blanket he's got (they were talking about the space blanket)!" They said, "I wonder how you can sleep comfortably with that wrapped around you?" And they would laugh and walk on.

I could not say that I had a fitful sleep. I felt I was sleeping, regaining energy, but there was a constant stream of these old people walking by the tree, staring down at me, making comments. Because I felt I was sleeping, I was not trying to contemplate what was being said, but there was some humiliation involved.

In my ceremonial tradition, I am not allowed to talk to people who have gone on to the Spirit World before me. In their spirit form, the dead people are ghosts, shadows of what they once were. I am not allowed conversation with them. It is just one of the warnings I am given in my ceremony, that that is not my job. Anyway, I felt a little humiliation with a lot of these comments, and a lot of support at the same time because there was jesting. There was humor always involved.

I slept at the sacred tree again on the second night, and nothing happened, I just slept. A cousin of mine sings the dawn song for the Sun Dance, waking the whole camp up each day. On that second night, I felt I was just comfortable, getting into my sleep when he started singing! He woke me up, but I survived for the morning of the third day.

I made it to the third day, which has the healing round. It is called the healing day. From the vision I had been given, the medicines of the Elk and the Bear medicine are my friends. I prepare them at Hollow Horn Bear Sun Dance every year to give to the people without fanfare, to help them. On this day, I brought the medicines out. I was unhooked from the tree to prepare and hand out the medicines. As I walked around the healing round to give the medicine to the people standing to be healed, I went through the round comfortably. When I finished my part in giving medicine to the people, I took my position back at the tree. The rope was tied back onto my pegs. I resumed dancing pulling tightly on the rope. I started praying again.

I was looking at the tree as the round was finished. I stood there in my position watching all the people go back to their places and watching all the dancers take their break. In the midst of this, suddenly, things started getting very dark. I was starting to lose consciousness, and I fainted. When I regained consciousness I noticed that I was lying face flat on the ground! I was breathing dirt in through my nostrils but smelled cedar smoke with its sweet scent. I became aware of these two young men fanning with eagle wing fans and smudging me with cedar. They did not bother to pick me up. One of them said, "No, we've got to leave him alone. We have to let him lie here because he might be having a vision!" I was thinking that this was a very hard way to do things. Why am I doing this?

159

I stood up after I regained full consciousness, and the singing started again. I started to dance. In the midst of this round of dancing, as I was pulling on the rope with my skin, praying and pulling back, a sudden gust of wind came from behind me. It hit the tree with force. The tree bent toward the west, and it pulled me forward. Trying to hold my balance, I moved with the tree. Then all of a sudden the wind stopped, and the tree sprung back. And I sprung back. Just as I was springing back another gust of wind came and again the tree went forward away from me. All of a sudden, the tension and pressure on my chest was gone. I looked at my chest. The rope with which I had been tied to the tree was on the ground. The pegs were on the rope. Instinctively I looked at my chest to see where the pegs were. It appeared as though the skin was still in place, that the skin had not broken, but it only looked that way.

Roy Dennis Stone, who was officiating the dance, came out to me, and he asked, "What happened?"

I said, pointing to the rope on the ground, "I don't know, the rope is there."

He grabbed the skin on my chest. He said, "Your skin's broken."

I looked again at my chest. "Oh, it is? What do we do?"

He said, "Let me go talk to the old people." He went back under the arbor as the dancing stopped, and the dancers were taking their break. A while later, Roy Dennis again came running out to me. He said, "The old people said they saw you being released by the Spirit People. You don't ever have to do this again!"

I looked around me. I had been dancing next to my brother Wesley, who was doing the same thing I was doing, dancing for four days. Since I was released, I knew I did not have to finish the dance. I took my pegs off the rope, and I took the end of the rope to the tree. I wished my brother well, and I walked into the arbor. I sat down. I said to no one in particular, "I don't have to do this again." My cousin and my uncle laughed.

One of them said, "I guess you've been let go. You don't ever have to do this again."

I learned what adversity meant. Even in the worst of times, when you connect with Spirit, you are released!

12

Hear Me! I Am Speaking for Them!

Iwayeceye!	I voice for it (Spirit)!
Namanh'un ye!	Hear me!
Iwayeceye!	I voice for it (Spirit)!
Namanh'un ye!	Hear me!
Iwayeceye!	I voice for it (Spirit)!
Namanh'un ye!	Hear me!
Iwayeceye!	I voice for it (Spirit)!
Namanh'un ye yo!	Hear me!
Maka sitomniya,	All over the earth,
Hoye wayeceye!	I send my voice for it (Spirit)!
Namanh'un ye!	Hear me!
Iwayeceye!	I voice for it (Spirit)!
Namanh'un ye!	Hear me!
Iwayeceye!	I voice for it (Spirit)!
Namanh'un ye yo!	Hear me!

As the spiritual leader becomes aware of the Spirit People, this song is sung to let the people know that the Spirit People are preparing themselves for communication with our world. The one at the center also is now ready to communicate with the Spirit People. Here the holy man has to let you know that he is now speaking for the Spirit. This is the affirmation that connects the material world with the Spirit World. You as a participant now must hear the Spirit!

The elders that I knew, in seeing their lives and in conversation with them as I was growing older, taught me one of the greatest lessons that I have found myself thankful for. In my life and its unfolding, the lesson that was great for me was learning how to handle adversity, exhaustion, or oppression, in any condition.

When you encounter a situation where you have used up all of your energies and resources, and you are being tested by that situation, the old people used to say that is an adverse time; that it is a very, very difficult time.

Christina told me that the old people who took on the ways of the Sacred Pipe and began to talk to Spirit People, and the Spirit People began to talk to them, had to learn how to deal with the most difficult as well as the most positive conditions. It had to be this way in order to speak appropriately with that Spirit World. Difficult times, times of adversity, exhaustion, oppression are the reverse of times when things are going well, when things get done appropriately, and things that are appropriately done lead to other activities that bring appropriateness and beauty.

Christina told me stories of the elders to whose ceremonies we would go. In particular, she used to talk about Grandpa Frank Picket Pen because his ceremony was the one that Uncle Leo sang at consistently and over a long period of time. She recounted, "Grandpa Frank is doing very well with his ceremony helping us, helping the people, and those who come to him. Often he reaches a point where he gets very, very tired and exhausted by all the people who come seeking help. There are times when he feels he cannot say no. But for him to get to this place, he used to always tell us that it took him nine *Hanbleceya* before he was given a vision to talk with the Spirit People. And on every one of those nine occasions, he was tested by the Spirit in some form—family going through difficult times, illnesses, deaths. You should learn from those people who have gone through things like that."

She said that when people are tested, these tests always come from places that you would least or not expect. They hit a person in such a way that this person can find no means or resources to deal with the situation. But if the person affected by these adverse conditions faces these difficult times and does things correctly, this person can get back on the path to doing things right and accomplishing good things for future generations. She would look at me with concern, then say, "Think of it this way. Grandpa Frank had to do a time of getting to know himself before the ninth try at the *Hanbleceya* before he was given the vision and spoken to. You should know that when a person is strong, this person meets this adversity. You'll find that they're happy despite everything that's happening to them. They use fun and humor," she would say, "despite all that is happening around them and to them.

"As you get older, you'll find that this kind of fun and cheerfulness with all conditions becomes a source for strength because it gives you stability that makes you rise above all the

165

things that the world is presenting to you. You'll find also that if you let your spirit be broken by these difficulties, you'll accomplish nothing—zero! But if you find that these difficulties give you new knowledge, wisdom, and the situations only bend you without breaking you, you'll find a power within yourself of rightness, goodness, and love. That's bound to manifest itself as doing things right and doing things in a good way, and that will overcome all those things that you encounter. A person who rejects wisdom and good things cannot make things right. A person who becomes great brings good and gets away from these difficulties to the appropriate path, because this person also knows that these difficult times will pass. When these difficult times are upon someone, everything that is done is not affected by goodness or love, and so one has to act good and be loving despite these difficult times."

She said, "I used to understand these men being in situations where they're denied, and their words have no effect. What you learn from them is that in these difficult times, it's important to regain strength within yourself, act in a good and loving way, and stop talking so much!"

I would ask her, "Why are you telling me this, because I have no interest in sitting in the center talking for people to the Spirit, and in turn, the Spirit talking back to me for the people. I don't have an interest!"

And she would respond, "It's good to know these things because if you do, you know that you have to deal with the good times and the bad times equally, but life is difficult for many of our people. It's just that when you hit these difficult times, as you will in life, those difficulties will exhaust you. They'll sap your strength. They'll take away all the things you need to meet those difficult times, so you have to go deeper into yourself to gain that strength that's always there. There will be difficult times for you. That's fate; that's the way of all people. So when life gives you a test and challenges your very being, you have to understand that you can do nothing during that time except to accept that difficult time and begin to be true to yourself." She would wait for me to give her a cue to continue, and I would give her one. She said, "And this means you have to go to the deepest part of your being. When you find yourself in the deepest part of your being, you'll find that all things that hit you, good times and bad times, are all things outside of you. You can still find joy and happiness within."

I would say, "That's very interesting."

"You have to understand," she would say, handing me some coffee, "that just like Grandpa Frank, when your goal is to begin to understand the Spirit World so that you can speak for them back to the people, you use up all the spiritual energy that the Spirit keeps giving to you. You use it up completely! You are at the place where life has to test you to see if you've learned those things that the Spirit World considers important in the truth. It's even more important that when difficulty first comes to you that the strength you find in yourself be used to overcome that difficulty within yourself. Doing this may not change the world around you, but you've overcome the trouble within yourself. If you are weak, the trouble will overwhelm you. It will overcome you, put you down. So what happens is, you fall deeper and deeper into self-pity, dark moods, and no activity. You begin to do nothing," she would say. "And all that does is make your troubles more and more hopeless. So it's best if you want to get back to a connection with your world in a positive way, you have to change how you think about those difficulties. You must change your attitude because if you don't change your attitude, you'll be deluded by all that you have to overcome, and you'll think that you have to overcome everything all at once. That doesn't lead to happiness!

"But if you find that happiness within yourself, that adversity, that difficulty that you are encountering, only makes you realize that you have to have joy and happiness with your relations, friends, and the world around you. And you begin to deal with your difficulties one trouble at a time. That will lead you back to honoring your friends and your relatives in a positive way. You will regain that sense of joy that will make everything move more to a point of resolution."

13

Send Your Voice!

Hoye ya yo!	Send your voice!
Hoye ya yo!	Send your voice!
Hoye ya yo!	Send your voice!
Hoye ya yo!	Send your voice!
Tunkasila!	Grandfather!
Eya yanka yo!	Say this as you sit!
Ikce Wicasa,	Natural man,
Ta Canunpe ki,	His pipe,
Le yuha hoye ya yo!	With this, send your voice!
Hoye ya yo!	Send your voice!
Tunkasila!	Grandfather!
Eha pelo!	All of you said!

This song is sung for the ceremonial participants to prepare themselves to have their request, prayer, or say in the ceremony. The word usage is exhorting those praying to use the wisdom and connection of the holy man to make their pleas to the Spirit and to *Tunkasila*. There is an assumption here that those praying do have a need and require some help from the Spirit World.

Christina shared many things with me about praying in the Pipe ways. She showed me how to make tobacco ties and how to use them. She also taught me what colors used with tobacco meant in prayer. She convinced me that praying in times of need was quite all right to do. Praying all the time, according to her, was even better. She often felt that people waited much too long to pray, they usually waited until things were really bad. When she was thoughtful about these things, she would take the occasion to tell me those things about which she felt something needed to be said. Once, I found her thinking out loud, "There are times in life, where there's no difficulty or trouble that's hitting you from the outside, but you find yourself feeling weighed down by the common things of life. When this happens, you have to stop and take a good look at how you relate to your relations and to your world. In that situation, everything outside of you is okay. You're loved, you're supported, you have food, you have water, but you're exhausted by all the things you think are common. So, you trap yourself into a position where you think there is no escape. When you find yourself in a situation like that, sometimes people offer help because they see you in such a dark place. People come to offer you help by asking you to help them. They ask you to help them because they may be facing difficulties, troubles, obstacles. You have to remember that you, yourself, are in that dark place. It's not good in that situation to jump into helping others to try to get away from your own problems. It's important to look at life and realize your dark place. Start to pray, start to make offerings to the Spirit World, the invisible world. If you begin to help others to forget your own problems, you may bring disaster to yourself and to them. You might not be wrong in terms of what people believe about good things, but because you are not in the right place to bring good things, your help could lead to disaster."

Another time, I walked in on a conversation between Christina, my Grandma Mary, and a Lakota grandmother, Susy Red Feather. Grandma Susy was a feisty older woman who was very knowledgeable, wise, and gifted in spiritual matters. She loved to wax philosophical with my Grandma Mary, and on occasion, with Christina. When I walked in on this conversation, they were talking about difficulties and adversities, real and imagined, that were affecting relatives of ours. My Grandma Mary was saying, "In a situation where you're only facing disagreeable occasions, that's the best time to learn to be patient and to wait until you get back into the light in your own view of honoring your relationship. If you can't do that, you go to a ceremony, regain a little sense of yourself, a sense of your own well-being."

I learned from their conversation that difficulty seems to be part of life, but just a part. There are ways to deal with difficulty. Often, when we face difficulty, it makes us restless, makes us indecisive, and so we push ahead. We want to keep pushing ahead. Because we are not in the right place, with very little energy to do the right things, it makes us deal with our troubles and obstacles in a very reckless way. We find that we cannot move forward, and oftentimes we cannot move backward, because we put ourselves in that dark place. It is as though we run into a door and the door will not open. We want to keep pushing it, but we think the door has got something against us, so it will not let us through. We try to figure out how we are going to get through the door without using the handle. We try to kick the door down, we begin to think of ways we can do this. All the things we can think of have no stability. The more we think of doing the wrong things, the more they become dangerous for us because we are leaning on them and they cannot support us. When we remove ourselves from the world in this way, all of our relations tend to fall away for that time, so it leads to great disappointment.

172

꧁

"I think it's very important," Christina was saying to Grandma Mary and Susy, "to try to stabilize yourself when you encounter trouble or difficulty. Because if you stabilize yourself, you will know how to look at things that work, and the things that don't work. But if you're not stable, it seems to me that you would endanger your life. Even bring disgrace to yourself. You can hurt yourself and other people. Even die in the process!"

I took from this that it is important in this journey inward to regain your strength, and also that you must begin to identify that which is stable, that which is strong and has proven to be strong. It is important not to break the foundation of that which you need to do. Grandma Mary threw in her comments to the other two, "So, is it like this? Is it like trying to put a teepee up with good poles instead of weak ones? Because if you put up your teepee with weak poles, that teepee will fall apart and injure you while you are inside thinking you have done something good. So it seems to me that it's important, when the world comes at you this way, to step away from the world to face the difficulty. Because the difficulty is happening, you need to step away to regain a sense of yourself so that the things you lean on will be strong and will support you. It seems the only thing to do where you can truly regain yourself and help others because that is the right thing to do."

Grandma Susy looked up at me when she realized that I was there. She turned her attention to me. "*Takoja,* when you do a *Hanbleceya,* to get to know yourself, that is one of the ways that you challenge adversity; you challenge fate, only to be able to accept things the way they are, good times or bad times. And, once you see that the Spirit World has accepted your offering and your sacrifice, there's still work to be done. Now we talk about weak people doing these things: what if you're doing well? What if you are in a high position in relation to the rest of the world around you?"

Grandma Susy said, "Remember, among the Lakota, that the leaders and the chiefs often are the poorest people in the tribe. Because the responsibility of their position requires that they give away constantly to their people, their sacrifices assure that the people will benefit and that their people will live. And in turn, the people support their leaders, but the leaders do not hold a position of wealth because they must always give. That is the way of our people, if you are in a position in life where you are doing well, you see the need of other people. Maybe you'd like to help, but instead of hurrying and putting energy where there's a need you begin to stop, you begin to hesitate. And you begin to count how you're going to help, it brings a lot of troubles! What happens is, those in a position to see and know what

173

you're capable of, take you away from that which you see as the need to help the people who really need help. They pull you into their circle, into their influence. You'll find that you'll have to do as they do, and you get stuck there. You can't withdraw from them. This leads to great embarrassment because what you had intended to do is not done, and the need of the people is not met. That's very embarrassing!"

Grandma Susy motioned to me to come closer to her. She continued, "But if you go back to your true goal of helping the people and those in need, the trouble you find yourself in passes very quickly. And if you really have an intention to do good and to help where help is needed, this offsets the mistakes you make and you are given your opportunity then to truly help the people.

174

"Helping the people can be very dangerous sometimes," she was saying, "but if you understand that your goal is to help in the places you can help, and you know that, you'll find that truth works for you. Sincerity works; honesty works. You'll find that if you're truly honest with those around you, and you're helping them, good things are already in your heart. So, it awakens the goodness in those others whom you want to help. And things get accomplished in a good way."

Grandma Mary chimed in, "So when you're confronted by difficulties and people pull you away from helping with those difficulties, if you go to your heart you will always understand what has to be done, even though you might be embarrassed for a time because you ran away from the responsibility. And if you, from your heart, know what to do in the situation that is the problem, Spirit gives you the natural opportunities to act in the way that will resolve those troubles, those difficulties. It's only important that you're thorough in addressing what has to be addressed. Don't get caught up in the dangers and difficulties of being stuck there. This requires great, great honesty with yourself. Those individuals who go to do *Hanbleceya* over and over to get to the point of influence with the Spirit World are confronted by this need to be sincere, to be honest, and to know how to face difficulties. What they learn, as I have seen them over and over, is this way of being honest. All the fancy things you do in ceremony to pretend to talk to Spirit World are dropped away. Only the simple things and sincere effort works. So, what they learn is that, in difficult times, you want to understand something; you want to help other people understand something. You learn through a *Hanbleceya* that you always begin with that which is the clearest and most understandable. You begin your journey from that point."

Christina jumped back into the conversation. It seemed as though I had become the focal point of their conversation. She addressed me, "Sonny! Now, if it takes you a long time to regenerate a connection within yourself, you have to realize that often we have the good of others in heart. Even having this goodness in your heart for others can be challenged when the world around you offers no help but only offers difficulty, problems, troubles, obstacles. You find yourself going for help among the people whose duty it is to rescue those in need when you find the world doesn't respond to you in this way. You have to know how to stop yourself. Again, make offerings and prayers to *Tunkasila,* and take the little things that begin to be good and harmonious. As you take those little things, you find that the world begins to take a turn for the better. It always happens this

175

way. But until things get better, this is what doing ceremony and praying does. Until things get better, you turn to *Tunkasila*. You regain yourself, you compose yourself. While you pray and offer sacrifice for the goodness and well-being of others, you begin to remove the obstacles within yourself, and you learn how to deal with them, what is the best way to maintain the good."

Grandma Susy seemed to jump onto Christina's wagon, because she pointed her open hand at me and said, "You must learn how to return to loving and good acts without losing yourself. This is done by delivering yourself with determination from those things that are weak, bad or small, or inferior, from within yourself." She dropped her hand in a waving gesture.

"The world around you is made of bad people, or weak people, or deceptive or manipulative people. Sometimes you'll find that they cannot be driven off by words or even by action. So the way to get back to your own goodness is to break completely in your mind from them. When you are truly sincere in your own mind that this is the way you want to be, you'll find that those people see that in you. They withdraw without your ever fighting them or encountering them." And she said, "If it takes your grandfathers and others many, many times to get a connection to the Spirit World, and they put themselves through all this difficulty and trouble to get that, you have to remember that Spirit itself has a role in who it wants to converse with, and who it wants to use as the doorway into this world. And it happens that sometimes it takes awhile for you to get to know yourself. The Spirit World waits for you to get to know yourself before it will come and speak with you. And when that time is appropriate, the Spirits will come. You will know that they are coming, and you will know that you are speaking for them because you are speaking also for yourself. At this point, you'll find that any problem or difficulty you encounter is like a big story." She chuckled as she continued, "Because if you know yourself, and you know your relation to the world around you, the Spirit World knows this also. You know the Spirit World and as you begin to know it, all those troubles you face begin to fall away. But because you still look at life as difficulty, you're undecided, you're uncertain, and you think that if you move forward you are going to make mistakes. But if you understand that you are now being given a way to deal with your own troubles, you know that these can be overcome within yourself. You can get over the mistake of not doing anything to doing the right thing."

Grandma Mary reaffirmed the words of Grandma Susy. "If you make a start in the positive direction with this knowledge, good always comes of it. So, when you're beyond your difficulties, there's always a step you have to take where you realize that that which has exhausted you is no longer present; only your mind is bonded to the past difficulty. So it's probably best that you get over the distress of it, and have some resolve and determination to remove that conflict from within your mind to help people overcome their own conflict. And get over that condition that you were in before. Have confidence. Mistakes from this point can be fixed. So if you grasp what's going on at this point beyond the difficulty, this confidence, changing this mind state to make a firm decision to do the right things, the difficulty is no longer a difficulty. And if conflict is still present, you learn to put away conflict because if you gain anything in conflict, all you get is more conflict."

Grandma Susy reached out and touched my shoulder. "If you think that you can gain advantage over all others by conflict, and you carry them to the end, you gain victory because you've won the conflict. You might for a time be praised for this, but your happiness will never last. Because in winning conflict, you open yourself to attack over and over again. That leads to conflict without end."

Grandma Mary was chuckling along with Grandma Susy. They had me in their grasp! Grandma Mary jumped right in where Grandma Susy left off. "So, if you overcome troubles by an acceptance of the conditions exactly as they are, good times and bad times, you overcome the bad times by proper action, by putting away your anger. Instead of being spiteful about your situation, you learn to accept things exactly as they are because these tests always come from the outside. They don't come because you are a bad person. They don't come because you did something wrong. There are just times in life when difficulties and troubles arise because others create them. And when you've used up your spiritual energy, and you're challenged and tested by this, these are the things to remember. You can master the test if you always come back to the proper attitude. Accept what you can't change, but grasp what you can change and make the decision to deal with it. In this way, all difficult times are overcome. When you reach the end of your life, and if you can die in your sleep," she was saying, "that's the best way to go. If you lose your life fighting, your spirit won't be happy because you'll have conflict without end."

"So these are things," Christina said, "that I, too, learned from watching Grandpa Frank." She then named some other grandfathers and grandmothers she knew that went on many vision quests to get this connection to the Spirit World. And I understood from her and my grandmas the meaning of the Lakota word *Tehiya*, which is difficulty or challenge. Even the greatest points of exhaustion, tests, and difficulties of life can be overcome by what you do with your mind and your action.

When you begin to acknowledge the Spirit within yourself, and that you truly are Divine Spirit, and you have a relationship with the greater Spirit that finds expression through your thoughts of goodness and loving acts, the greatest difficulties are mastered. They are overcome. That lesson has always stayed with me.

Christina often reminded me of the stories about Grandpa Frank and other men's *Hanbleceyas*. She said, "The other thing you learn from these older men who went on these *Hanbleceyas* to get a blessing from the Spirits, to speak for them, is that if you really do want to connect in this way with anything, you must persist with this action. You must stay focused on that will you have, to do these things. You do it until the Spirit responds. And remember, all you get is more responsibility to do more of it. This is what is difficult about life, and also challenging. You can look at it as difficulty, or you can look at it as challenge. Then, you are free to live your life till the end of your days. These old people have gone through a lot. I'm sure that they're leaving much for you to learn and handle for the rest of your life."

179

14

Greetings!
I Am Eagle Thunder!

To live the way of the *Canunpa,* the Sacred Pipe, according to the elders, is always a sacred, challenging, and oftentimes difficult thing to do. Especially when you enter a relationship with a Spirit friend at the altar, the work becomes even more challenging. I have been given an altar and a Spirit Friend to work with in ritual and ceremony. The Spirit that comes to the ceremonies that I conduct currently appeared after what seemed as an evolution of four spirits that frequently visited us in ceremony. Those four were First Eagle, Lone Eagle, Little Wind, and Big Loud Thunder. They would normally appear individually at the Eagle Ceremony that I officiated. I am not certain that the Spirit that comes to the ceremony now, Eagle Thunder, is truly a combination of those previous four, but that is what seemed to happen at the time Eagle Thunder first made its appearance.

In the Eagle ceremony, the first two Spirits I was allowed to speak to came as a result of a ceremony that I had asked for as a *Wopila* (an appreciation, or thank you) in Denver, Colorado. This happened in 1979, at the home of my *Hunka* brother, Tom Teegarden. Many good things were naturally coming to me at the time I requested this ceremony.

I was employed as a program analyst with the National Indian Health Board. One of my responsibilities as an analyst was to research and find ways and means to unite health practices of native traditions and the Indian Health Services, Health and Human Services Department of the federal government. What I was finding in my studies and analyses led me to fully appreciate the sacred ways of our people. I received many wonderful blessings from the world in support of that. For that reason, I wanted to say a thank you to the Spirit, as is the tradition of our people, for those blessings and good fortune that were entering my life. I wanted to do this in a sacred manner. So I called my uncle, Charlie Kills Enemy. I asked him if he would conduct a ceremony, a *Wopila,* for me. He agreed. I called many of my friends, cousins, and other relatives. I asked them to be present for this appreciation ceremony that was to be conducted for me. I called my uncle, Wallace Black Elk, to come and help.

In the ceremony, conducted by Charlie, several things happened. First of all, Uncle Wallace and I were given almost an encouragement, a blessing, to take our spiritual ways out into the open—much akin to being given altars. Then my Uncle Charlie said in Lakota to me, "First Eagle and Lone Eagle are going to speak with you." What I thought was a simple *Wopila* turned into a little bit of an "inner adventure." I was experiencing a sense of dread about the responsibility of taking on an altar. But because the situation transpired as a movement of Spirit, I was confused and bewildered. I was speechless, yet feeling awe and wonder at the same time.

As I was hearing the gift of an altar from the Spirit World to work ceremony, I was also being given four cautions, or warnings. I could take an altar out into the open to work with people. I could help them in matters of will, of the laws of nature, of looking into the future for potential decisions, and of helping them to heal and see the promise of better ways to live. All of this had to happen from a point of disinterested truth that could lead to sharing the joy and pleasure of living.

It has been many years since I have come to understand what those meanings were, but the cautions I was given were pointed. I was never to use a ceremony for personal gain or purely to make money. I could get gifted by those who asked me for a ceremony by any means, including money, but I was not to do them as a conscious effort to get money. I was not to use a ceremony to wave my banners nor to market myself as a healer, medicine person, or holy person. If others saw that in me, that was of their own choosing. I was not to take that position to market. Secondly, I was not to use a ceremony or spiritual ritual to curse people or to use negation to harm or injure another being. Thirdly, I was not to talk to Spirits who experienced life before. This meant that I should not talk to anyone, including my own relations, who had made their journeys into the Spirit World. I was and am not allowed to use the *Hocokan* for that purpose. And the fourth caution was that since this way of Spirit is open to everyone, to all colors, I was to be honest

183

and sincere in whether I could help an individual or not. If an individual asked me to conduct a ceremony on their behalf for healing, blessing, or to get any of the information that I was allowed to ask for, I was not to use this ceremony to do what I could not do. In other words, I was not to say to a person that I could help them if I could not. And the direct caution was that if I could not truly help a person, I would always have to refer them to someone who could, which is information we could find through the ceremony.

The cautions that were given showed me the way to conduct myself. Since then, I have learned how all individuals should grow and develop in a path of their own choosing that reconnects them to the spirit within, to the spirit without, and to the consciousness of life itself in all matters of being.

184

The Spirits that first came to talk with me when I experienced them were unbelievable. Aside from the teachings of the elders and people that I grew up with, I had been trained to look at life rationally through the schooling I had had. My formal education came through the Todd County Independent Schools District in South Dakota; Lenox School, a private college prep school in Lenox, Massachusetts; Dartmouth College in Hanover, New Hampshire; Harvard University in Cambridge, Massachusetts; and several other colleges where I had taken courses of study. Through those institutions, I was taught how to study rationally, reasonably, and supposedly realistically. I was to do this all the while maturing with a cosmology that looked at life as the co-existence of the Spirit World and the organic, material world. This has always presented me with a paradox, a dichotomy, and a challenge as I was going through my education. I knew that I really believed one thing—yet I accepted another. I found myself at odds sometimes with what I was learning rationally, but also knew and accepted spiritually.

By the time I arrived at Dartmouth College in 1969, I had encountered a spiritual tool of great significance in my life at the Minneapolis Airport in Minneapolis, Minnesota. In the fall of 1968, I was returning home to Rosebud, to bury my brother Joe. He died from injuries as a result of a car accident that happened just south of St. Francis, South Dakota. Four others had died in the same accident. When I heard that he had died from injuries in the accident, I went into a deep state of anger, disbelief, and grief. On the way home to South Dakota from Lenox, catching a plane in Springfield, Massachusetts, I was truly grief stricken. Having a dread of flying, I imbibed too much alcohol. I was too numb to make a clear choice about anything. Landing in Minneapolis, I headed into the astrology section of a bookstore in the middle of the airport. As I walked between rows of bookshelves, I unintentionally bumped into a shelf. A book fell at my feet. It turned out to be the *Book of Changes,* the *I Ching.* I picked it up and began to read the first writing that my eyes fell on and encountered a spiritual experience that has stuck with me from that time to this day.

As I read what was on those pages in the *I Ching,* the Sage, I realized that I was reading a description of my immediate situation in metaphor. Metaphor is a descriptive process that my own Lakota language uses. I was, through the fog, amazed and frightened by that experience. I closed the book, put it back on the shelf, and continued on to the astrology section where I distracted myself.

I arrived in Rosebud in the evening of that same day. During the wake for my brother, I found myself very angry at the Spirit World, angry at all my relations who allowed this to happen. As I indulged in this anger, I encountered some hard and clear teachings from the elders about how to deal with death, life, birth, and life beyond. As I was being talked to, lectured, and directed, this tool that I encountered at the airport—the sentient Sage in the *I Ching*—seemed also to stick in my mind as one of the "Old People," one of my elders. It became a study of mine after that.

Many things I have learned of the Tao and my own growth and development within the Lakota tradition have resonated with each other. In my own acceptance of the cosmology of the Tao, I have arrived at a point in life where I have to look at truth simply for what it is, using the language of the Tao, the vision of the Lakota way, and my own insight. Perceiving my life in this manner has been very powerful. I have gained a tool with which I can look at and accept the movement of all that is as it is in the world we live in. In using this tool, when I was introduced to the Spirit World through the ceremony in Denver with Uncle Charlie, I already had a language which helped me to begin to understand at least some of the metaphor and symbology that was being presented to me by the Spirit World.

I thought I was in good shape since I had a language to understand the Spirit World. The actual experience of communicating with the Spirit People while in the state of rationality was, on the other hand, quite a shock. After the initial gift of the altar through Uncle Charlie, I fought with myself. I truly questioned whether I actually had the right to do these things. Was I just playing a mental game for my own ego's satisfaction? Was this gift of the altar truly from the Spirit World? Was *Tunkasila* really asking me to offer my life to serve the Spirit's needs to save the people?

One of many things you learn in ceremony about working with Spirits is that it is a reality that no one else around you, near you, even those who believe in Spirits may experience while you are in contact with them. So it gives to others in the rational view a sense of you, the healer or medicine person, going through what appears as a schizophrenic or psychotic experience. When in this state of communication with the Spirit World, however, I was told that you should never lose sight of yourself. In being taught the ways of the ceremony that I now do, you must maintain yourself. You stay in your own center. You must accept and use, through song and through vision, what the language and communication of metaphor and symbol is telling you. You must stand between this world and the sacred world, the worlds that exist side by side, to know the important things that balance both worlds.

187

Over the years, in the process of overcoming the inner struggle, several Spirits, presented by the Spirit World as true helpers, have shown up in ceremony. Of the Spirits, Lone Eagle came first. First Eagle came second. Then a little wind spirit, named Little Wind, impish and playful, occasionally visited. Then the first experience of *Wakinyan,* Thunder Spirit, followed. Its name was *Wakinyan Hotanka,* which means Loud or Big Thunder. I always heard through the teachings of my elders that when you encounter Thunder Beings, you have to deal with the *Heyoka* (Clown) part of your nature, being contrary, and looking at the realities of life backward. And yet, the encounters I had with the *Wakinyan* Beings simply said, "You must work with the *Heyoka* people. Do not consider yourself a *Heyoka* (because I would have trouble doing things backward)!" That may in itself be backward!

An *Inipi* I was conducting at the home of Robert Jacobs in Taos in the early 90s proved to be a life-changing event for me. In previous ceremonies I had conducted, the four Spirits would show up from time to time. Sometimes, they would appear inadvertently, but always correctly. Appropriately, they would come into the *Inipi* lodge. On this particular occasion they all appeared together, one at a time. Not one word or vision or symbol was given, but they started to swirl into one image of a great being. In my mind, from this swirling image, I always had the image of these four Spirits becoming the one Spirit that I now work with. But I'm also certain that I am confused about that reality. The Spirit that spoke to me after that event told me in the language that it spoke that it was sent by *Tunkasila,* that it was a Thunder Being. It was sent to have a relationship with me.

The Thunder Being was sent to be my buddy in the spiritual realm, not because of the backward nature that I exhibited, but because through me, *Wakinyan* (Thunder) would reach the world. It would help the world find a new period and development of growth that we all must prepare for. This new time of growth would begin to happen after the millennium year in change. We happen to be in that time. (I do find it of great personal interest that we are now writing this book—"we" in the sense that others are helping with this particular writing, both from the material as well as the Spirit World.)

So, this Spirit came into the lodge and said in Lakota, *"Hau le miye yelo! Wakinyan Wanbli le miye yelo!"* In English, "Hello (or greetings), this is I. Eagle Thunder is who I am." And then, it proceeded to set down the formality under which we would speak. We were not allowed to speak to each other except in ceremony. Or in broad daylight and during ceremony it will appear as image, a voice, a loud wind, or a loud sound. The situation must be appropriate for both of us. I was not to lose my center nor go into a trance, but be in conscious communication with a Spirit whose role it was to help the world. Sent by *Tunkasila* to give message, to convey, to foretell, and to work with medicines that were to be given to me. I had to be willing to be its partner, its counterpart in this world. I agreed.

Since the time it appeared in the early 90s at that ceremony, Eagle Thunder has always arrived appropriately at most of the ceremonies that I have conducted. Very few times has Eagle Thunder not shown itself to me. When there is a no-show, I have learned to look at it not as a break in communication, but a time when there is no need to connect our two worlds.

In this ceremony that I am doing with you, the reader of this book, imagine as we have entered this part in the ceremony that you encounter certain lights in the darkness. You may see lightning bolts in the darkness of the room. Or you may have no phenomena at all, but you sense a presence, an energy. You are not going crazy! You are experiencing a change, a shift in energy, vibration, frequency. No matter how you might describe it, you sense a change that all of a sudden occurs. And then, you hear me at the center of the *Owakan* begin to voice for the Spirit Being.

189

The Spirit enters and says, "*Hau,* I am Eagle Thunder. What is the matter? Why are we here?" And so, in Lakota or in thoughts, I say to Eagle Thunder, "I am High Star, your friend. I have a relationship with you. I intend to ask you those important questions of life for which *Tunkasila* has sent you. The questions I wish to ask you this day come from people who wish to know what healing is. They wish to know the healing ways of the native people on *Unci Maka* (Grandmother Earth) where we live. They want to know not only practices, but what is done in healing. I can share with them what I know, but I wish to share also my discussion with you on these matters. So I will ask these questions: What is healing? What is Native American healing? What is Lakota healing? And what is my healing?

"I will ask you, 'What is my healing?' And I will ask this not in terms of ritual and process in the world, but for my own journey of self-healing, and I will share this also.

"Let us begin . . . !"

15

We Talk of Healing

Eagle Thunder flashes a symbol first and shows me thunder. Then it shows thunder itself being supported by the gentle wind. Thunder, being itself, gets louder and gives more energy to the gentle wind. They begin to support each other. I am being shown union between these two forces, a union that appears to last a long time, personifying an enduring condition.

"Thunder and wind always show up together." Says Eagle Thunder, "The wind is gentle by nature. The thunder moves all things by energy and shock." Eagle Thunder goes on, "The situation that I describe by image represents an image of union and commitment, like the lasting union between the male and the female. This union is represented by forces that can come together, but must hold together by will, where the moving force directs and holds relationship from the outside in, while that which is gentle and yielding by nature holds from within. So the relationship builds, supports, and moves the two forces together."

I say to Eagle Thunder, "That is a rather confusing image at the moment!" I ask, "What am I to tell those who wish to know by written word, or by image, or by metaphor, what you are telling me?"

Eagle Thunder says, "If anything is to have a lastingness, something that is to endure for a long time, that leads to the coming together of all that is beautiful in a successful manner, this coming together must not incur any blame or fault. Once this uniting occurs, holding together must be accomplished with great persistence. It must have a direction. It must have a place to go!"

So I say, "What do you mean by anything that is long lasting?"

Eagle Thunder says, "Anything that lasts long has movement that is not worn down by obstacle, by obstruction, or by hindrance. Anything that lasts long is self-contained and self-renewing. It is a movement that is firmly organized. It is a movement that is integrated wholly in accordance with all that is natural in law and beginning new movement at every ending that it completes." A silence, then, "Look at your life! Feel your body! What I am pointing out to you is much like the breathing that you do. As you take a breath, your body begins to pull in, to contract. When you can no longer breathe in, this movement turns into a new beginning, in which the movement of your breath goes outward from you. In your exhale, an expansion occurs. This is the movement of your life that tells you that you are alive. Stop breathing, and you do not last very long!"

192

Eagle Thunder flashes an image. "Look at the heavens above you. Everything that you see in that sky moves in a path that is fixed. All the bodies that are there appear to give light. This has been going on long before you. It will happen during the time that you live here, and it will happen long after you are gone. This is what the Spirit People mean by that which lasts a long time. In the world around you, four seasons are in motion. They follow a law of movement that produces effects that show you long lastingness. If you as a human being want to find a meaning, to embody a lasting meaning in your way of life, you must be as dedicated as those four seasons. Thus, your world finds form from your many experiences. If you want to understand the nature of things including you and I, of all that *Tunkasila* presents and all that *Unci Maka* presents; if you must understand it, look at what gives those things, those beings in the skies above you and on *Unci Maka,* that which gives them long lastingness. You will then begin to understand what gives them the laws of their being. The very things that make them what they are. Look at thunder, look at the wind!"

Eagle Thunder continues, "We give you these pictures because the law that makes the wind, the law that makes the thunder, shows their extreme ability to move. On the surface, this law does not look like that which lasts a long time, but it is the law. That which makes their appearance, and their going away, the coming and going of these very forces endures beyond the flashy showings of wind and thunder itself. And so in life, if you as a human being wish to have long lastingness, you must learn how to stand firm. Stay in your direction and purpose until you have completed them. And if what you do is completed, you begin a new one. A new way."

I ask, "What does this mean?"

Eagle Thunder rumbles, "Look at the forefathers before you. Look at who you share life with now. Look at the children who are coming behind you. If you wish to know the independence of that which is idealized in life, the growth of that which is high cannot be based on the rigid and the unmoving. All those who came before you, all those who share this time with you, all those who follow you, all face the law of having to change with the times. Or, the times will come and shatter the rigidity. So, what has to endure is the very nature of that which gives life to those who have come before you, to those who share this time with you, and to those who will follow you. This is what endures. Every end is followed by a new beginning. The new beginning has an end that leads to another new beginning. If you act always within that which you understand, that which coincides with what endures, that law of your being, that nature of your being, if it determines all of your actions, you will live a long time."

So I say to Eagle Thunder, "What you are telling me is that the laws, the nature of things, determines how things last in our world?"

There is silence. There is a flash of light. Eagle Thunder booms, "Look closely at that which lasts a long time! You must understand that in the time that you now live, the effect of time is the quickness or the hurry with which lastingness is attempted. Haste in attention and the stress of that haste to create an enduring condition is rarely achieved in your time. It is a time of tension, a time of restlessness. This uneasiness has become the enduring condition of your times, and so it constantly brings the opposite of that which is good. Look at the world around you! It is composed of individuals who live in a state of constant hurry without ever attaining inner composure, inner calmness, inner tranquillity. This is the sickness of your time. This haste, this restlessness, not only prevents thoroughness but becomes the greatest danger when it becomes dominant in places of leadership, of authority, of knowledge, and of wisdom!"

So I ask Eagle Thunder, "What is this leading to? I asked, 'What is healing?' You are giving me these many images about long lastingness!"

Eagle Thunder responds, "In order for your time to understand independence, interdependence, sovereignty, the understanding that must be gained is that your world must nourish that which is appropriate. Body, mind, spirit, these must be all nourished equally. And if you must nourish equally, you must prepare the food, cook it! In order to cook, you need the flame, the Spirit!"

So I ask again, "What is the teaching here about healing?"

With what sounds to me like a gentle blowing breeze, Eagle Thunder responds, "For your world to attain its proper relationship to all things living, for all things to have the consciousness, the mind of *Tunkasila,* this order, this way of believing, this way of being, must take up the new that renourishes that which is most appropriate. That would be the ultimate in goodness that your world can experience, that would lead to the gathering of all that is beautiful. When you have wood and you set a flame to it, it leads to nourishment, because it is the flame that cooks the food. So, to give nourishment to the Spirit is to live those truths exemplified by sacredness. Those who are holy, who

195

have touched *Tunkasila,* have touched that which is. It is done in a sacrifice where all that is visible has an effect of that which is good. What is good must grow beyond itself into the realm of the Spirit World, and find a true blessing there. Along with clarity, this goodness must take firm root in the order of the world as that which is being acted upon and lived. That will be the new, the sacrifice to live that which is good. This is what will bring the world back to order. This reaches beyond the culmination of civilization as you know it. Not only in religion, but in the way of action, in the way of spirit. Serving the sacrifice of goodness serves creation, for it is the true sacrifice to *Wakan Tanka,* the closest relationship that you know and must reconnect with. That which is held the highest among all that is living must be acted upon and given back to the divine. The divine in turn does not manifest itself apart from life. The supreme visions, the revealing of *Wakan Tanka,* appear to the holy people and to those who see the future, because they know the laws of how things work. For every person to venerate truth in the holy people and in themselves is a veneration of the Great Spirit. The will of *Wakan Tanka* (the Greatest Spirit) is revealed through those who have followed the holy path, the sacred path. If one accepts this truth as a way of balance in life, a healing takes place. The forces of life take their proper positions. Those who are healed in this way have inner light, and experience understanding that allows them to accept the world as it is. This must lead to the greatest good and the coming together of all that is beauty. For humanity to find the proper healing, it must put its fate in proper order by making its position correct in relation to the rest of life. In human life there is a fate, there is a destiny that lends power to

196

life in its expression. If humanity succeeds in assigning the right place to life and to fate so that the two come into harmony, fate has a firm footing in the appropriate. For human beings, it means to take care of the body. Nourish it well. Take care of the mind, give it knowledge. Take care of your action, give it wisdom.

"So, if you wish to know that which always is, that which lasts a long time because it simply works this way as a matter of law, know what abides always. Know what to do to return to a correct place. And if you move things to a correct place, there is a firmness that develops around its expression. A human being can have many, many experiences without ever being overrun by those experiences. So, they unify the expression of the nature of that being. So, 'What does lasting a long time mean?' It means that in thought, look high. In action, act within that high view, but with understanding so that adaptability and action work together to give a sense of lastingness in time. If you wish to correct things, persist in the course of correction until it is complete. The heavens above you, the earth below you, they endure, they last. They will go on for a long time! Why? Because they act within their nature, and things come to be as they are.

"When you achieve something, let the completion of it lead to a new beginning. For that person who wishes to correct the course, to balance the forces in one's life, that person must learn to remain forever in that course of correction, balancing. Bringing one's forces back to the right place in the world, one can reshape oneself to completion. This is the nature of *Tunkasila* and *Unci Maka* in all beings. That thought in action and the understanding from this imparts a lastingness both to the action and to the thought. The meaning here is that the conditions for

197

that long lastingness and its necessity consist in that persistence in the correct course. Being persistent, giving continuity to change, is like a plant that grows from a seed, achieves duration, flowers, beautifies itself, and drops another seed. The secret of the universe and its eternity is the endings and beginnings that compose the lives that find expression in it. In the world of human beings, being persistent in a course of action leads to the goal. The end is achieved, as completion is a short development that occurs. A new beginning is joined with another end. If you move much, you must rest much. The rhythm of all that happens is a relation of motion and stillness. So, in human condition, if you stand firm in the correct course, do not change your direction but stay within it to its completion. When you go with a movement in a course to its completion, long lastingness is achieved.

"In order for a true healing to take place in the cosmic order of your time, those sharing your time in life must learn a process of taking up the new—they must have a transformation. And in the world that you live in, there must be a correct way to reorganize the social order to meet that which is appropriate; nourishment of the spirit, action in spirit, and goodness in the world. That action must be mutually reinforcing of all that is appropriate and good. This is the only way that sovereignty of being can find appropriate expression. The correction of your time, which is to calm restlessness and stress, is to reorder the social organization so that spirit prevails. When true sovereignty is exercised, fate is placed on a firm footing that honors spirit and sacrifices in action, goodness, to its finest expression. This is what is meant by putting fate in its right place by making the position correct.

"A healing occurs when all the forces find their proper place and are expressed through thought and action. Life must be kept light and burning with truth in order to attain a condition so long lasting that the sources of life are constantly renewed. This applies to all of human community and institution, relationships and positions; leadership and authority have to be so regulated that the order created finds long lastingness, endurance in that which regenerates goodness. In this way, fate shows where leadership and rulership is given in the most appropriate way so that others can be helped along to that point of duration, long lastingness. A healing is a correction of force and a renewal of life at every turn."

I say to *Wakinyan Wanbli* (Eagle Thunder), "I'm not certain if I quite understand yet what you're saying to me. It will take my thought and contemplation to come to this order that you speak of, and obviously the Spirit World is pointing to what it is showing me. But I want to ask you the next question.

"As I was asked to write this book about Native American healing, I ask for the Spirit's view of Native American healing. I have already stated I can only address a part of it which relates to my own experience. So, in turn I ask you, the Spirit, what is Native American healing?"

I hear laughter from Eagle Thunder and a loud sound, a movement and shake from the sound of thunder. I see an image of the sun shining over much movement, much "busy"ness. I am also shown the image of a mouth wishing to speak but something is in the way of the mouth—perhaps it is full—so no sound or garbled sound is heard from the mouth and its lips. It becomes obvious that the lips of that mouth cannot be joined because there is so much in the way. Then, I am shown a storm. There is much thunder and lightning. There is a disturbing tension that is created by this apparent awesome movement of weather over plains that were once calm.

The people in the image are moving about in constant hurry. There are figures in what appear to be military uniforms who are grabbing people, and tying the people with ropes and chains. The tied and shackled people are being thrown down in front of judges. The judges are judging, throwing penalties at these individuals who seem to have created disharmony. The judged seem, also, to hold no care for order or truth especially from the mouth in relation to the world around them.

I look at these images. I look at them very closely. And I say, "*Wakinyan Wanbli,* what are you showing me? I asked about Native American healing."

Wakinyan Wanbli says, "What the Spirit World is showing you is to make you aware of a growing danger. This danger is related to what is known as Native American healing and its coming to the marketplace. The business and the constant motion of those under the sun, bartering, haggling, trying to find a price, are creating an obstacle to the truth of the balance of life and the practice, the being of life. There is a need to bring that which is just to correct the whole situation. This is not a view of healing, it is the selling of healing that does not allow truth to find expression in proper ways. What you are seeing is this: Truth and that which balances, and their necessary union, is being obstructed by talebearing. By deceit, by interference, and by falsehood, many through the marketplace are blocking the way to a union of knowledge and activity that can bring long last-

200

ingness to all of life. The laws and energies of life are priceless—
they merely exist for the expression of life.

"Any obstacle to that union of wisdom and action must be
removed in order that the gathering of beauty and its necessity can
happen appropriately. The Spirit World shows that permanent.
injury can happen to those who are given half truths to follow and
live by. The union of truth and action is divine. Any person who
follows the false, or is misled by the false through seduction, cannot find the divine. To prevent that, there must be measures taken
to bring truth and wisdom to a proper acceptance in the order of
life. Obstruction that is deliberate, placing price on wisdom and
healing, does not vanish of its own force. Judgment, activity, punishment are required to remove this deliberate obstruction, or at
least to deflect it. But even that must be done in a correct way.
There must be clarity. There must be enthusiasm for truth. The
clarity must be yielding. Enthusiasm must be tough. Too much
hardness, too much excitement, would be too violent to mete out
correction. Lack of clarity and lack of adaptability is too weak in
energy to make the correction. But the two together, mildness and
firmness, can create a just and middle way whereby appropriate
decision making can be taught to humanity. This will find gentleness and respect. It would be appropriate for any individual to find
ways of activity, laws, and policies that clearly define penalty for
that which is done incorrectly, wrongly, or badly. The law should
define and specify just penalty. If both mild and severe penalties
are clearly differentiated according to the nature of the wrongs
committed, clarity and order begin to appear in the social order.

"Clarity and severity in appropriate punishment to the
breaking of law has the effect of instilling respect, not intimidation,

201

but respect for that which must create order. Penalties are never ends in themselves. Obstructions in the social order of humanity increase only when there is a lack of clarity in the penalties and slackness in their execution. When there is only a slight application in the execution of just penalties, disorder necessarily arises. The only way to make strength for the law is to clarify it and to make penalties appropriate, certain, and swift, to the nature of the crimes."

Here again, sitting in the center, talking to a Thunder Being, thinking that I am going to receive a direct answer to my question, I seem to be getting a lecture on law. How am I supposed to apply what I am experiencing to arrive at clarity about Native American healing?

So I ask Eagle Thunder, "Does what you are giving to me mean that Native American healing is inappropriate?"

And again I hear laughter from *Wakinyan Wanbli* (Eagle Thunder). "In the old days of your people, the Lakota, the elders knew how to hunt game, kill the game appropriately for the needs of all to be met. The meat from the game was dried on a high place so the animals could not get at it, and the birds were kept away by someone watching the drying process of this meat. It became a way to make nourishment last a long time. If you gained merit, you gained reward such as eagle feathers, or gold. But anytime that you had a reward for the merit that you gained, it was because you became aware of the dangers of the position that you had attained."

I am bewildered. I remark to Eagle Thunder, "This is bewildering. It is, at this point, not registering in my understanding. It does not make any sense to me."

Wakinyan Wanbli continues, "Anytime a situation of right or wrong is perfectly clear, but cannot be decided easily, there is a tendency for human nature to become lenient. That tendency leans to being soft on that which has to be decided in order to make merit and reward appropriate to the activity that has occurred. To receive something like yellow gold is a symbol to be true and impartial, to follow the mean in justice. To remain true and impartial, one must remain conscious of the dangers that can grow out of the responsibility anyone assumes to be correct. In making a correction, one must also avoid making any mistakes that intentionally harm the good order of that which can last. What is meant here is that in the human realm, one has to make one's activity follow the law of creation and to make oneself innocent, make oneself guiltless, and put away guile.

"When a mind is natural and true—not shadowed by reflection or ulterior motives—and the nature is directed by spirit, truth and innocence are restored. When one gains conscious purpose without spirit, a degenerate nature begins to build. Truth and innocence become lost. So, in order to make a correction with great clarity in appropriate action to move to order, purification must take place. Things of beauty are brought together by purifying that which is impure, and by consistency in that activity of purification.

"Good only arises naturally in your world when one is as one should be. And if one is as one should be, true direction is created by following the nature that is innately good that guides and should guide all of one's actions. This is a gift from creation. If one is devoted to the divine spirit within oneself, the purification that occurs can lead one to do correct and appropriate

203

action with certainty, with confidence that goes beyond instinct. Devotion to the divine spirit within oneself leaves ulterior motive and thought of reward and personal advantage behind for the gain of all life.

"The kind of certainty that brings about the unity of beauty and that which is appropriate can only be furthered by consistency, by persistence. Only that which is correct and appropriate and in accord with the will of the Spirit World, *Tunkasila's* world, is good, affordable, and available to all. This quality of correctness, of righteousness, must have proper reflection and forethought of action to bring that which is good. The Spirit World in blessing supports this. When the Spirit World does not go with one's deeds, one's actions, it only shows one's departure from purity and innocence. And that which is not good becomes the lot. So all things can attain the natural state of purity if action is undertaken appropriately to meet the demand and duty of a time. And by action in harmony with that time, all beings high and low are fostered and nourished.

"If one wishes to lead others to do that which is right, one must always draw on the spiritual wealth of life, and take care of all forms of life. One must respect and honor all forms and ways of living, do everything to further them at the proper time. The state of goodness and purity always brings the supreme happiness of the unity of beauty and long lastingness.

"This is what is seen as the picture of all the truth taught in the native traditions. The truth is in all native traditions. It is not in only one. The direction given as a whole in the native traditions is to return to a nature that has forethought and proper action to be as one should be, with the healing forces in balance and harmony with time and its demands. This creates a union of perfection and beauty. And as ideal as this may be, it is what comes through the purification process in your world. For instance, among the Lakota, striving for purity in the *Inipi,* to find the breath of life, is such a process. In all of native traditions, this purification as a process is always available, but it is not available through price and marketplace. That is what must be corrected to understand what Native American healing really is. Native American healing is about a life-giving process. It is not a consuming process. So it cannot be correct in the consumers' world."

I laugh, because I thought Eagle Thunder made a pun! Or at least I understood it as one! As I listen to Eagle Thunder, I realize that I am unclear yet as to the meaning intended by the images I am receiving. I decide to take a different direction.

I inquire of Eagle Thunder, "Well, if that is Native American healing, then what is Lakota healing?"

Eagle Thunder is silent. There is a low rumble, then quiet again. Next, I hear a booming sound. What I hear is unusual to me. "Among the Lakota, the balance of life occurs when fire clings to water, and water clings to fire. They embrace each other delicately. When a transition from confusion back to order is complete, and everything is in its proper place even in detail, you can be led to believe that this is extremely favorable. Be careful! Give thought to this! When perfect equilibrium enters any situation, any movement within it can cause disorder equal to the order just achieved. Lakota healing, in that the fire is clinging to the water, and the water is clinging to the fire, presents a condition of dealing with times of climax that require the utmost balance. This shows the necessity to exercise the greatest caution

205

and precaution. When anything reaches order in the highest sense, the only gathering together of beauty that can be brought in union occurs in small things. Even then consistency, persistence, are needed because anything that finds the ultimate order begins in a good way and always ends in disorder."

So I say to Eagle Thunder, "What does this signify?"

Eagle Thunder says, "Everything is in a transition from the old to the new time. It presents a difficulty to that which is old and no longer useful. And it presents a challenge to that which is new and is just beginning to be useful. Everything that your people need to know to practice and to share with the world stands in proper relation to the world. So, truth can be taught as well as learned. Beyond the forms, traditions, and practices of your people is a life force that touches and exists in all things. The Lakota people have been touched by *Tunkasila* to express their part and gain knowledge of this in their own ways. To the extent that the Lakota people wish to share their part of this life force there is a perception of things coming together successfully. So, there must be care that appropriate and correct attitude be learned and taught. Everything in your world will proceed on its own accord. This is dangerous because it will tempt those who are lacking in caution to relax and let things take their course without troubling over details. This will lead to an indifference that is the root of all evil. Decay can only arise from this indifference. But even though this is the course of history in anything that comes to its completion, it is not an inescapable condition or law. If one understands this, one can avoid its effects by great persistence and extreme caution. In the Lakota world, knowing how to balance the forces is a process of beauty. But to achieve perfection in balance requires the greatest caution to maintain that balance. So, for the best in the Lakota culture to find expression in life, looking ahead, thinking of the bad things that can happen, can arm defense against decay far before its possibility of expression.

"This is what is meant by water clinging to the fire and fire clinging to the water. All of life in those two elements stand in relation and generate energy creating the tension of life. This tension demands caution. Too much of one thing harms the nature of the other. So, if one understands these elements in relation to each other, one understands that their generating energies are hostile to each other. So extreme caution can prevent damage. Through a process of ceremony and ritual, the Lakota people can find themselves at those junction points when all things are in balance and work in harmony, so that everything seems to be in the best of order. But it is only wisdom to recognize the moments of danger and know how to prevent it by means of taking the necessary precautions.

"Lakota healing, as well as all other forms of healing, will be needed tremendously in the near future. The world is moving into a time that needs to be faced with care. The times that are evolving will show revelation of greatness as well as create great scandal. All culture is entering a time of flowering but in that flowering, a convulsion is bound to happen, uncovering hidden evils within societies. So they cause great sensation. A time of balance, because it is favorable, presents a danger that these kinds of evil can be easily covered and concealed, so everything is forgotten. And the illusion of peace complacently rules. To those thoughtful individuals who hold the way of life in practice and

207

in mind, these occurrences will only present grave symbols that cannot be neglected. If those who are watchdogs for goodness prevail, they will find and present the only ways of averting evil consequences to humanity. And so, Lakota people are in a position to show where these evil consequences can occur and be of use to humanity in this way. But once this is evident, Lakota culture and all that it has to share and teach must present its good side, so that the way of behavior and conduct of governing all people becomes a choice of change to action on the spiritual truth. Since Lakota people as a majority do not hold their own way as sacred, it will fall to the holy people of all cultures to attempt to unite in this way of harmony. When others accept this, the beauty of truth, not only as a Lakota way, but the truth of all ways will have its own day. The actions completed to this end will show that which is to be believed. And the success of it, to the consistency of those who practice peace and harmony will help to remove all cause for mistake.

208

"In simple terms, the greatest changes in personal behavior and political upheaval are possible in the coming, immediate times. They will become necessary, but even then, they should be undertaken only under the greatest necessity when there is no other way out. Those who must change this way must do so when confidence of the social order is gained, and they are called to the task. That can happen only when the time is correct and ripe for growth. Then the procession to the completion of the task must be done in the correct way so the people find joy and enlightenment to prevent excess. What is needed for every individual who follows the sacred path is to free oneself of selfishness and relieve the need of all people who need spiritual truth and guidance for the self-healing that must take place. When this happens, there will be great rejoicing in that which has been corrected.

"Times change, and the duty demanded by them changes also. In the world cycle, there are winter, spring, autumn, and summer of the life of peoples and nations. These call for the greatest social transformations to do that which is correct.

"Lakota healing and all other healing must know how to deal with the demand and duty of the time to remove that which is a great sensation from scandal and to put all forces in their proper perspective and balance with the greatest caution. What this will begin to show is that only in this way can all humanity master changes in nature, by acceptance of their regularity and the processes in which this regularity occurs. Order and clarity when understood remove chaos. When humanity understands this it can adjust itself and advance to the demands of the different times that are unfolding. This is seen as the healing process of all things which include the Lakota."

I ask a final question. "Eagle Thunder? What is my healing?"

"A gentle wind blows freely in the sky. The power of that which is small often restrains. It can tame or it can impede. Look west. The promise of a great, nourishing rain begins to rise in the west. You see it. It is still in the west. The greatest strength in your being is temporarily held in check by a very weak element. It is by being adaptable with this knowledge in your action that can lead to appropriate outcomes.

"So, what does this say? The moment of your greatest influence is yet to come. You can show the people a promise of a better life, a promise of a better time. But the moment for

209

action in any sense cannot arrive yet. So, disinterested truth in working with any individual becomes the key ingredient to leading people to a state of healing. When you know how to share true joy, you know how to share pleasure with another in the most appropriate and enduring conditions.

"Pleasure shared in living life becomes pleasure doubled. In your personal life, when you cannot have great influence, even though your power is strong, learn to refine your nature in the smallest ways so you are not obstructed by the greatest weakness of others. If you exercise your strength and adaptability, your strength becomes centered and your will is done. This leads to success. The power that is evident in the nourishment that is coming in the storm can go further than what you believe that it can go, but the influence has not yet set in. So apply inner strength with an outer gentleness. This is the greatest and easiest way to your achievements yet to come. Center your mind and your will is done."

Eagle Thunder! I am groping. "Does that mean that I have yet to have great influence in the world?"

Eagle Thunder says, "You are building influence. You have promise to show the world what it needs to know."

"So what does it mean by refining my nature in gentle ways?" I ask.

ET (my affectionate acronym for *Wakinyan Wanbli*) says, "Your understanding can penetrate everywhere. That means refinement. But you must follow the way of the holy people. This means exercise the essence of your being, your character. Let clarity guide you. Let refinement find expression in living out the fundamental principles of your life. Without drawing inappropriate attention, you can counsel others in the greatest truth from a disinterested position. This can help them make the decisions to find spirit within their own beings. You can help them with the spirit to find its greatest expression in their actions. And when you share joy, it comes through your understanding. Devote yourself to that which is good. Gain trustworthiness. Gain the trust of others in your behavior and your pleasure is doubled. In this way the greatest good can be achieved. The wealth of spirit, and the wealth of being, can find expression clearly with great strength, honesty, and kindness. This is what is meant by the promise of the nourishing rains coming from the west. Creative expression finds truth only when the will is in accordance with the truth of the spirit. If you do not understand this, it is time to work."

211

So I sit back, look at all the metaphors and the language that the Spirit World has shared with me. I ponder, "Is this the time to share what I have just experienced from the Spirit World? Are eyes and ears open, and thought, broad enough for others to see, to hear, to think and contemplate truth presented in an unfamiliar fashion?"

It is time to share this with those who use their eyes and thought to understand the symbols presented to me. Let the reader contemplate this meaning in a personal and individual way.

Much deception can be given in healing forms. Much truth can be given in healing forms. The greatest healing occurs when an individual decides to be as one should be. Healing forms help when weakness predominates, and the goodness and love of others lift the spirit upward. The actual healing occurs when one accepts the truth and sets life straight.

From my discussion with Eagle Thunder, I can reaffirm my position that there is nothing that can be justly called Native American healing. There are definitely healing forms within the Lakota, the Dine, the Hopi, the Cherokee, the Ojibway, the Comanche, and we can name all of the tribes still existent as having healing ways. Healing, in any form, must address the reconnection to Spirit and the balancing that must occur in that reawakened relationship. And I gather from the Spirit that living life is in and of itself the healing process! To attempt to gain healing from process in the forms, personal or judicial, will fall short of its goal and lead to great deception. To have the true healing, an individual must work to remove the obstructions and reawaken the spirit within.

212

I say to Eagle Thunder, "In this way, you have helped me. In this way, maybe, I have helped you, but I accept this relationship. I am complete in my communication with you. Let us be done." *Wakinyan Wanbli* gives a rumble, a couple flashes of lightning, great laughter, and there is silence.

My thought now is, "I have lived through this again! I laugh! I laugh as you sit in the ceremony with me. I laugh, not at you, not at your action, but I laugh because there is joy. Joy that there is great balance. There is great equilibrium. I learn, and keep learning each day that we must be careful even with truth."

We are not yet complete with our ceremony. You must understand that we now have to return this Spirit to its place and close the door. Whether this ceremony has helped you or not, now we can let the Spirit go and return our lives to dealing with the mundane. I hope you will once more rejoin life.

Looking back at what Eagle Thunder presented to me, I heard a prediction. Scandals affecting many in this world, including the Lakota, are presented. Will there be a scandal? If truth is not used appropriately, yes. Will it cause great sensation? I do not know. On the flip side of that, I heard of great discoveries and revelations coming. Will those hold true? Let us wait and see! Whatever the future may hold, what you have experienced thus far is a ceremony that I promised I would do with you. If you prayed during any time in this ceremony for your own well-being as well as for others for balance, the Spirit will help you, because that is your connection. If you have believed that I have done the healing for you, then you may certainly need to change your path.

213

16

I Give You Grandfather's Prophecies

Hoye
Tainyan,
Kinanjin pelo.
Hoye
Tainyan,
Kinanjin pelo.
Tunkasila,
Tawokunze,
Ca lena cic'u welo.
Hoye
Tainyan,
Kinanjin pelo.
Tunkasila,
Tawokunze,
Ca lena cic'u welo.

Sending their voice
Clearly,
They step back to their place.
Sending their voice
Clearly,
They step back to their place.
Grandfather,
His prophecies,
So these I give to you.
Sending their voice
Clearly,
They step back to their place.
Grandfather,
His prophecies,
So these I give to you.

This song is usually sung to signify that the Spirit has completed the communication with this world and has returned to its position in the Spirit World. In some ceremonies, this song is referred to as the *Kigle Wicayapi Olowan* (Sending the Spirit Back Song). The word usage conveys that the Spirit has sent its voice and has returned to its place. The word for spirit is omitted in the song. The implication is the reference to many Spirits having sent their voices and returning to their places. The references to *Tunkasila* and his predictions being given to us ties in the Spirit People to this return.

After my rebellion against my Uncle Jim at the Fools Crow Sun Dance, I had returned to the Hollow Horn Bear Sun Dance to help my own band, my own tribe. I had the intention of helping as I had been away for a long time. Years after having the vision at the Fools Crow Sun Dance, I had heard that my Uncle Jim had had a heart attack and was having open heart surgery at the FitzSimons Hospital in Denver, Colorado. Since I was still living in Denver at the time, I drove to the hospital, which is located in the eastern part of the city, to go to see him.

The doctors and nurses somehow knew that I was supposed to be there. Apparently, someone had told them that I was expected. I walked into the main part of the surgery department to look for Uncle Jim. I was directed by the nurse on duty to the surgery recovery room. When I entered the room, I noticed that it was very cool. I immediately saw Uncle Jim at the far end of the room lying flat on his back on a table and obviously out very cold. There was a sheet covering the bottom half of his body. The upper part of his body was bare. He had wires attached to his temple, his chest, and his arms. He had an IV going into a vein on one of the arms. He had tubes going into his mouth covered by an oxygen mask.

I walked to him. I touched him and said in Lakota, "I'm praying for you, *Ate* (Father), that this test and challenge is something you can overcome. And that my prayers, hopefully, along with all the others' prayers will help you." I leaned close to his head and said, "Besides, you wouldn't want to look like Robocop for the rest of your life (since that's what he reminded me of, with all those wires, and his chest being sewn up the way it was)! Then I chuckled, patted him on the head, and left the room. I spoke to the nurse about his condition. She told me that he was in critical but stable condition. Satisfied with what I heard, I left the hospital.

Among the Lakota, we learn to laugh at even the worst times and the worst conditions. We do this not to make fun of each other, but to share humor. One of the great foods of life from *Tunkasila* is humor and laughter. Laughter nourishes the soul. This is what I have also been told by many singers who shared song with me when we sang together. I shared a good chuckle with Uncle Jim.

A month after my visit to the FitzSimons Hospital, I came to the Denver March Powwow, a community gathering of all the Indian tribes around the country at the Denver Coliseum. This song and dance celebration is held in March, and has proven to be a grand celebration of song and dance. So I go to this event as much as possible because I sometimes have a role of speaking for the people during the event. At this particular time I was carrying out my role, speaking for the people in their giveaways and

217

social rituals. I noticed that my Uncle Jim had walked through the main entrance to the Powwow. After I finished my tasks, I went over to him, shook his hand, and hugging him I said, "You don't look like Robocop anymore!"

He laughed and said, "I heard that you had come, but I was away off in another land. I had this urge not to come back because everything was so peaceful there." He sighed, "But *Tunkasila* felt that I should come back one more time. It's good to see you, my son!" We laughed together and talked a little bit. He took on a serious tone. "I have a favor to ask you."

I responded, "What is that, Uncle?"

He said, "Since you left our Sun Dance, no one talks about peace anymore. I would like you to come back this summer. Take a break from your busy schedule. Come back and talk to the people about peace. And bring your medicines; I've run out of those things you've given me! I use them to help myself and the people around me. I ask this of you."

So I said, "Okay, I will come back to your Sun Dance this summer." We parted. I continued my functions and singing songs during the celebration.

In the summer, after I had finished my duties at Hollow Horn Bear Sun Dance, the Fools Crow Sun Dance was taking place on the following weekend. So I stayed in Rosebud visiting with relatives and my brothers. I went to Kyle, South Dakota, on the way home to Denver. Driving through Kyle, I went straight to the Sun Dance located west of the town. Once at the Sun Dance, I walked underneath the arbor to where my uncle was sitting. I brought him a fair amount of the two medicines that I work with. I gave them to him.

I said to Uncle Jim, "This is what you asked for. Anytime you'd like me to get up and speak to the people about peace, I will fulfill my word to you."

And he said, "Good." Just then, the *Heyoka* people were doing their ceremony. Pulling a dog's head from a boiling kettle of water, they were doing a healing for the people in the midst of the Sun Dance. The main *Heyoka* picked up the dog's head. He walked over and handed it to an elderly gentleman, one of the leaders of our tribe. As the elderly leader took the dog's head, he came and sat down next to me and Uncle Jim.

He looked at me and said, "Here's this young man who is very knowledgeable, very educated, knows a lot about the ways of the white world." He pointed the dog's head at me and he said, "But you are not Lakota." He continued, "You have stayed away from our people a long time. And your knowledge doesn't make you a Lakota."

So I looked at him. I was not uncomfortable, nor was I even moved by what he was saying. I responded to the older man, "I've learned from many of you that prayer, no matter how you do it, is the most powerful action you can take to connect with all people and with *Tunkasila*. I may not be a Lakota in your worldview, but I'm Lakota because I grew up as one. I will not defend that to you. It's just that I know what my life is and has been. I have a feeling that I know what it will be in the future." I quieted my voice. "If you are trying to upset me, please stop because you will only upset yourself. Besides, I'm going to live longer than you. If you think that I'm not going to have influence, I'll have it far more than you after you're gone (I admit that that was my ego statement to get under his hair, but I said it)!"

219

He again pointed the dog's head at me and said, "You do not fear the Spirit People. Be afraid of the sacred ways; they are dangerous! You should know they are dangerous!"

All this time he was pointing the dog's head at me. I thought, "Poor guy! (I was referring to the dog.) It gave its life so that the people would live. Here is this person using it almost as a weapon!" I leaned over to Uncle Jim and mumbled to him, "I don't think that dog likes being pointed at people!" Uncle Jim was trying to maintain propriety, as this elderly man was truly one of the leaders among the Lakota. Uncle Jim did not want to upset him. But he chuckled under his breath. The man got up and walked away.

220

Uncle Jim turned and asked me, "Did he upset you?"

I said, "No. We have this weird relationship. It goes back a long way. A lot of his anger toward me comes from envy due to singing. He's just carried it over to the sacred. I just think that's going to be a challenge for him to deal with this."

I then said to Uncle Jim, "When I speak about peace, I'm going to speak about what it means to be a Lakota, as I was taught growing up. Uncle Jim, I learned a lot from you, and so for you to ask me to speak about these things to the people, I will use this as an opportunity really to address peace. I have no upset about what this man has said, but I will mention it as a way to encourage our young people to continue to be Lakota. No matter how much criticism and degradation they receive from those who don't think we're doing it right, our young ones should continue."

Uncle Jim laughed and said, "Before you speak, I'd like to have you come and do a healing for your mother (he meant his wife, my aunt and *Ina,* mother) Florine." And he called her over.

I took her, and I put a skirt around my waist, and took off my shirt, shoes, and glasses. When you enter sacred ground, you remove all things that are metal or anything that has to do with impropriety, or not of the Lakota world. So I took my *Ina* out to the sacred tree. I prayed with her and helped her with a healing. I actually felt *Wakinyan Wanbli* enter the tree. A huge gust of wind came up, shook the tree, and touched my *Ina*. I finished praying. I said, "*Ina,* I don't know what the matter is with you that Uncle Jim would ask me to do this, but I have asked *Tunkasila* for a healing for you. I believe that *Tunkasila* has answered. You should just watch yourself so you can walk a good path." She agreed, and she gave me a big hug.

Uncle Jim came out to the center as soon as he saw that we were finished. He came to the tree, touched it, and he prayed. Finishing his prayer, he stepped back to stand by me. He was looking around the dance ground at the people. He looked at me and asked, "Do you know that you are *Tunkasila?*"

I looked at him, and I said, "What?" I was a bit surprised that he would ask that.

He asked again, "Do you know that you are *Tunkasila?*"

And I said, "In thinking about it, I think I know what you mean. But you'll have to be a little bit clearer in case I am misunderstanding what I think I understand."

Uncle Jim chuckled and continued, "You are *Tunkasila.* Why would you say '*Hau*' and agree, when in prayer, people address *Tunkasila?* You sit and you say, '*Hau.*' The moment you say '*Hau,*' you are *Tunkasila.* Everyone who sits in the center, everyone who comes to the tree and prays and answers as *Tunkasila* is *Tunkasila!*"

221

Now, in modern thinking, I understood that he was saying the Spirit is within us, the Great Spirit that is a part of everything. So I said, "I think I know what you mean."

He had a stern look on his face as he faced me. "Son, stop
thinking! Just accept that's the way it is. And if you know that,
your way will get more power and energy so the people can be
nourished." He said, "Look at the people around you. People
relate to each other either as leaders or followers. How people
behave, and how people act toward each other always changes.
When we touch the *Tunkasila* within, you begin to understand
that life that is given to us, that life that presents its needs is
always the same. This can't be changed. This gift that we have
from *Tunkasila,* life is all around you. It will never go away. That
life you have is no more or no less than any person, or any animal, or any plant that lives. It exists for one and for all," he said.
"Those who come before you, those who are with you now, and
those who will come, they are all meant to enjoy life in all of its
inexhaustible opportunity!"

"Hau!" I agreed.

He said, "There are two things you should know if you are
to have influence that helps people satisfy their needs in behaving well toward each other and in working together. These two
things go down to the very depths of life. If you and all others
don't meet these two things, human order, human effort, falls
apart. Now, these two things are very important for you to know.
You have to go down to the deepest part of life to know what
its needs are. You must work to satisfy those needs, or at least
influence the satisfaction of those needs. If you don't do that, it's
as if you have done nothing at all. Finally, you must teach the

222

people caution, care. Because if you succeed in teaching them carelessness, it only brings disaster. Every individual who walks here in this life, no matter how they might be different in their knowledge and in their personality, character, in the world, the foundations of our lives are the same. They exist in all of life!" He almost shouted, "Every person who has reason can think, can draw on the course of gaining knowledge and life from the depths of *Tunkasila*. You experience it in your own nature!"

Quietly, but with great intent, he continued, "So you have to be careful that you succeed in your quest for knowledge to get to the real roots of life and get away from those things that everyone else thinks, because if you think like everyone else, it's like having partial knowledge. Sometimes, it's like having no knowledge at all. You must remember to always keep working at improving yourself, because if you don't, you might collapse . . . like I did!"

He laughed and said, "Every one of us has this little man within the heart. We have to let this little man out to stretch in the world, to touch others, to embrace them, and to pull them in. Once we imprison this little man in the heart, we have things like a heart attack. I know, I experienced this one!" And he laughed again.

He turned to me and said, "So, *Tunkasila*, encourage people to work with each other and do all that you can to get them to help each other. Get them to do well in their work, whatever it is that they're doing. You are in a position of influence to organize others. Help them to cooperate for the benefit of all things they do and for all of each other. You'll live a long time if you do it this way." Then he said, "Come here." And so I went to him, and he gave me a hug.

223

We went to the tree, and he said, "When you step into the center, here, people see you. When people say that you have great wisdom, great influence, half the people will bow down before you and want you to save them. They will prove to be as bad as those who don't want to be saved. Which means that the other half will compete with you and tell you that you're not real, that you are not Lakota, that you are not a human being. They will try to put you down! But I want you to know something: When you look at the world around you and half the world is struggling to even realize its own goodness, it's like walking around in mud because all significance for life is lost. And this half will throw itself away. Expect to have a tough time with relationship by these others. Those who are walking in the mud are not asked for help or even given a hand.

"Look at them! If they maintain this walk of theirs, no one troubles about them anymore. Their task becomes one of learning how to be patient again. They look at the world in anger or aggression to try to have it their own way. They have to put up with the gossip that they incur by their own actions, and they have to put up with their own actions and their consequences. And so their task becomes one of having to relearn how to face things exactly as they are again and to be truthful with themselves, otherwise they lose their life. So," Uncle Jim continued, "you have to remember this when you stand at the center. You have to uphold the significance of life the best that you can. This means you have to have the courage to face things exactly as they are, without any deceit, without any pictures of how you want things to be but how things really are. In that way, you can address anything that you encounter. This recognition and understanding only gives you the opportunity to be firm and to be consistent in your action to bring things back to order. That way you can meet your fate, that plan that *Tunkasila* has for us, in a good way. All it takes is good laughter!" He laughed and continued, saying, "When you know this you can go out, eat and drink with your buddies, your mothers, fathers, aunts, uncles, grandpas, grandmas, and even the little ones, because you'll experience happiness and a good laugh. It's always important to understand destiny. If you understand destiny, you don't worry about it. You don't try to shape the future by interfering in things before the time is ripe anyway. So if you understand that things will always change, and things always give you new pictures to look at, you'll understand destiny and fate. When it comes you're ready. It just means to know what you know and hold onto that which lasts. Keep things simple. Lead a regular life; don't try to impress the people because your being in the center already is attractive to many. Don't waste your strength! Keep yourself free of mistakes for as long as you can because they become sources of weakness. So if you understand this, you'll know that there are times when you are truly doing good things, but people don't make use of you because they're still working out their issues.

"Know that there are times in which danger appears naturally. Danger appears when you know you are a good person, you have good qualities, but you begin to neglect them because the world around you doesn't seem to accept them. And it happens because no one bothers about you. And if you let it get to you, you become weak in the mind. You deteriorate. And so you turn to the weak people trying to do something worthwhile, and you cannot because you haven't given yourself the strength to know that even in the best of times we can run into trouble.

"In those times, always come back to the holy people. They'll set you straight. But also know that if you do choose the good and no one bothers about you anyway, you shouldn't worry about it. In those moments you have to learn how to accept your own goodness, your own capacities. Purify yourself. Time will come when people will come to you. At those times you'll wish that they don't come because it can get pretty busy. So it's important to understand this. Just like when you didn't want to talk to *Tunkasila,* and He talked to you anyway. When you're in danger and you face the weaknesses of others," he said, "try not to escape it all at once. Learn how to wait. Learn how to deal with the disagreeable situations until you see a way through those dangers. You'll know, truly, how to protect yourself. These are ways we must learn as we stand in the center, sit in the center, and we speak for *Tunkasila* to the people. So that's why I call you *Tunkasila,*" he said. "So, *Tunkasila,* learn this well!"

I stood looking at Uncle Jim for a little while, since we were in the midst of the Sun Dance. One of the challenges of being at the Fools Crow Sun Dance is its location. The dance is held in a little bowl area, surrounded by buttes. On top of the buttes, because of the breezes that hit them, it can be five to ten degrees cooler than the dance ground. But at the bottom, that little bowl where the dance is, temperatures can exceed 100 degrees with no breeze. So it can make you feel as though you are in a kettle, cooking, and being cooked. Standing next to Uncle Jim after he called me *Tunkasila,* I began to notice how hot it was out there on the dance ground. I also began to notice how the sun was beating down on our skins, and I was feeling the discomfort.

He again looked at me and said, "When you overcome your difficulties, especially at the point of overcoming your difficulties, you have to learn to let the world go. Learn to face it alone, learn to renounce all those things that people hang on to as 'the way.' Put all of those things aside. You must become like a stream of water that all life can come to of their own free will and be able to drink from. The water you present must be drinkable. It must be nourishing." As he mentioned water, I began to get thirsty as I was experiencing the heat of the sun even more.

"So there is a time when you have to sit back and let the world go by so you can clear yourself, you can purify yourself. These are times when you work to put yourself in order. When you're putting yourself in order, you can't really do anything for others. But the work you are doing is truly, truly valuable because by enhancing your abilities, your influence, your knowledge, your wisdom, you set yourself to be able to help others and to accomplish those good things after this period of purification is over. It is stabilizing yourself, putting yourself on firm footing, so that even if floodtime waters come and wash everything else away, you're standing firm. Your stability has allowed you to survive the onslaught of not only people, but of events that you have to deal with. So always remember that when we turn to the Spirit World and acknowledge *Tunkasila* within and without, we still have to do the good things. And if you're doing good things and people learn from you how to do good things, you learn that people are then drinking from your waters." He pointed at all the people in the circle. "All leaders in life should give power to their words by the actions that they undertake. They should understand and translate the good things and loving things of life

227

right back into life and understand that it is a step-by-step process. The good things do not all come at once or overnight. They come step-by-step. If you are there providing water, nourishment to all, no one's forbidden to take water from you, to take nourishment from you, except those who by their own nature or by their own attitude cannot be nourished by you because you cannot help them. But it means that you should always be open so people can drink from you.

"This truth that you express will be a great blessing to life," he said. "You must have the courage to do good and great things. Your inner self, with its life, is inexhaustible in this way, so the more people draw from you, the greater the gifts *Tunkasila* gives to you. And in this way, you can work at helping people remove decay from their lives and decay from your own life. And if you truly follow the ways of *Tunkasila,* there are points in life where you don't serve the needs of those who govern people. They come to serve their needs to you. That is not a powerful position. It is a responsible position. It's good to remember that you don't serve them. They come to serve you so they can in turn nourish their own, those who follow them.

"And there are times when you must do something that is not for humanity, but for yourself and for all of life. These things are good to know," he said. "It's a way to reorganize your life and learn to truly help those who live to work properly with great help to each other. You can learn to help them in this way."

Though it seemed like a long afternoon (when I look back on the time we spent out there), we were no longer than an hour standing in the center. He was saying all of these things as a lesson to me. In one instance, he was chiding me for rebelling against him, saying that I should pierce so I could talk to *Tunkasila*, and on the other, pointing out to me that my rebellion led me to having to pierce anyway. In the Lakota, piercing is an act of rebirth because when you split your skin, and you put a peg in it to hold the rope to the middle of the tree, that rope is called *Cekpa,* which means umbilical cord. When you break after having done this, you are reborn. It is a way of the warrior tradition to overcome one's ego by humiliation of the ego, so that one can regrasp and have an understanding of life again. This rebirth lets you live again.

And so, in this time period, much later than that rebellion I had, this is what Uncle Jim said to me in the center of the circle when he came and asked me to speak about peace. A little while after our talk, I had the opportunity to speak to the people about peace.

229

17

I Give These to You

Cic'u welo!	I give it to you!
Cic'u welo!	I give it to you!
Kola!	Friend!
Wayanka yo!	See it!
Cic'u welo!	I give it to you!
Cic'u welo!	I give it to you!
Wounye wan,	A cloth banner,
Wakan ca,	Is sacred, so
Cic'u welo!	I give it to you!
Heya,	Saying this,
Hinanjin a u welo!	They come to stand here!
Kola!	Friend!
Wayanka yo!	See it!
Cic'u welo!	I give it to you!
Cic'u welo!	I give it to you!

Canli wapahta wan	A tobacco tie
Wakan ca,	Is sacred, so
Cic'u welo!	I give it to you.
Heya,	Saying this,
Hinanjin a u welo!	They come to stand here!

In this song, the holy man and the participants in the ceremony are giving their offerings to the Spirit World. These offerings are usually the tobacco ties, the cloth banners, the sacred objects, and spirit food that were needed to conduct the ceremony. What has been used as well as that which has not been used are offered and destroyed after the ceremony. The word usage shows that the people stand to give up that which has been offered. This song is then actually an offering song for those tools and those gifts which you have brought to the ceremony.

"I give it to you, I give it to you. Understand what it is that I give to you." The understanding is not about the material, cloth, tobacco ties, but again it is a saying that one recognizes the Spirit World as being present in the moment that you are also giving your offerings. The song reaffirms this reality.

When I spoke to the people at the Fools Crow Sun Dance upon Uncle Jim's request of me to speak about peace, I recalled that in growing up, many old people and many of our own contemporaries would always say we were not Lakota. I related the story of the event that had just happened a couple of hours before, when this elderly gentleman had confronted me about not being Lakota because I and others were not doing it the way Lakota people do things. Based on my grandparents' and my uncles' and aunts' teachings, I realized a truth about our people,

232

the Lakota. The Lakota people are a group of rugged individualists. The challenge for them at all functions that they undertake
is to unite as individuals in a common purpose, a common bond.
The language that we speak together fortunately connects us in
communication.

The traditions of song and dance that we celebrate help
us to connect to a far greater reality that we are intrinsically a
part of, but separated from by our own thoughts and actions.
And because the Lakota people are rugged individualists, there
is a healthy competition, as well as an unhealthy one, amongst
individuals as to who is doing things correctly or not.

All of the teachings I had received up to that point in my
life told me that all of us as individual Lakota would be driven
to do things our way, as individuals, first. It appears that our
lessons have to be directed toward how we could put aside that
individual character for unity of purpose with others. If those
lessons are successful, we might find that we could accomplish
great, good, and loving feats. As I recounted that, I said that every
elder who has ever sat down with me, and every contemporary
man or woman who sat with me and said to me that I was not
Lakota, each of them taught me a different way to be a Lakota.
So at one level, they must all be correct. Or they are all wrong.
But in learning that, as I have grown, I have also realized that all
of us, no matter what culture, no matter what tradition, no matter what race, we truly have a human foundation that is the same.
We all do the best that we can to give expression to what the
ancestors have left for us. We also do the best that we are able to
do from what we experience in our present life to bring those
truths that we learn about life to manifestation.

233

I have learned from every one of those individuals that unless we offer our beings, by giving power to the words that we speak, by action; unless we really truly offer them to creation as an expression of that which we are, we bring disaster upon ourselves because we then disconnect with the spirit.

As an individual, no matter how much criticism or blame becomes attached to you, the challenge as well as the difficulty of living that gives you opportunities to unite with others in a common purpose that is good and that is loving should be accepted and undertaken with great energy. I have understood from many ceremonies and from my discussions with the Sage that peace is complete. It is complete in that utter state of union, harmony, unobstructed blending of energies of the strong and the weak, the light and the dark. All things truly gain life from this contented blending of forces.

As I have worked throughout the years in the healing traditions, I have experienced the truth that every human being is given the opportunity to express life peacefully. In sharing knowledge and wisdom with those who have come to the altar with me, with those who seek an understanding of the future and their part and their will in it, I always point out that the striving for peace can be dangerous. The danger of our times is that people look at peace as a state of utter calmness, tranquillity. I find that peace itself is the most dynamic condition in life that furthers the well-being, the goodness, and the production of further life in its expression. And yes, tranquillity is involved in peace, but it is not peace. Tranquillity is tranquillity, calmness is calmness. Peace is dynamic. And so I said this to the people, "My Uncle Jim has asked me to come and speak to you. To talk to you about peace.

Apparently since I left here to return to my own people to do work over there, no one has talked of peace here."

Between the Sicangu and Oglala (Rosebud and Pine Ridge), because of the common language and relationship we have (we used to be one tribe at one point), there is a constant teasing, a constant putting down of each other. I had the urge to dig deep into myself and bring out some Oglala jokes. I bit my tongue and realized that this is an opportunity given to me by my uncle to speak to the people about a far greater need to recognize, to understand, and to express peace in life. Peace is an opportunity truly meant for us all. It is difficult for many to get to peace because the wants, the desires and the passions are the very first things that one draws up from one's own mind.

I shared this with the people. When I finished speaking, I said to Uncle Jim, "I thank you for giving me this opportunity. It makes me believe in peace; that it is available to us all, and that the world truly needs it at this time. But it must start with every individual who consciously knows that peace is peace, and that it is what brings growth, development, and prosperity to life. The truth of this is evident only by its expression in those things that occur."

Repeatedly, my people have pointed out to me that after times of great difficulty, after times of great challenge to one's own being, we have to reorganize our lives to be able to help life along to a better path. If we truly understand that we have to take our knowledge of how things work, how united work achieves great things, and to teach these to the people, we will endure as a human race. In teaching the people, we have to constantly influence and exhort them to help each other. If they do not know how to help each other, it becomes an individual

235

effort again. Great purposes are not always achieved by single individuals. Even the person who becomes holy, the person who really connects within his own soul and being to the sacred, has had help along the way. This is what Uncle Jim and many of the other individuals who sit at the center, sing for people, and talk for *Tunkasila* have understood. They have taught this to me and my people. This truth comes from antiquity. It must find its expression in our present. It must continue onward. I believe many of my elders knew this, so they taught it to those of us willing to learn, without shame or attachment. This is just the way things are. This is the way things work.

When I came back to the Hollow Horn Bear Sun Dance to offer my being to *Tunkasila,* to the holy people, to the Sacred People, and to those who need help, I did it with an understanding that we truly are protected by a force far greater than ourselves. This force does not control us, nor does it have direct authority over us, but it finds its expression through the lives that give expression to truth. The sacred is expressed and conditioned by human life, and that is the only way we know it as living beings.

236

18

We Watch You from Above

Tunkasila,	Grandfather,
Lehapi k'un?	(Remember) you said this?
Letanun welo!	It is this way a while!
Ninwankabya,	Above you,
Awaniglak'	We look after you,
Unk'un pi ca,	Being this way, so
Taku otehika	Whatever is difficult
Wanicin ktelo.	Will be no more.
Ehapi k'un?	(Remember) you said this?
Letanun welo.	It is this way a while.
Ninwankabya,	Above you,
Awaniglak'	We look after you,
Unk'un pi ca,	Being this way, so
Taku otehika	Whatever is difficult

Wanicin ktelo.	Will be no more.
Ehapi k'un?	(Remember) you said this?
Letanun welo.	It is this way a while.

This song is popularly known as the *Woawayanke Olowan* (Protection Song). Many song men who have shared variations of this song with me said that if this song is sung in one's worst and most trying moments, *Tunkasila* helps immediately to overcome the difficulty of the moment. The word usage shows that *Tunkasila* here is looked upon in the plural sense as connected to all that was before this time. From high thoughts and views, everything is protected. This protection continues for the while that it is called upon. And because there is a promise by *Tunkasila* for this protection, the song asks *Tunkasila* to remember this promise.

As one of the closing songs, this song says to *Tunkasila,* reminding *Tunkasila* and all those who came before us, that they left these truths for us. It has been this way for a long time. We acknowledge the spirit, not in the literal, material sense as above us, but with that understanding and clarity of a high view. These truths, these understandings, and wisdom are made evident because they can be seen clearly. If we apply these truths and wisdom of life to our present action and manifest them in this life, no matter what difficulty befalls us, there is always a way to get beyond it. The difficulty becomes no more when we understand this. I believe this to be a teaching of all traditional peoples in the world. All spiritual walks say the same thing. It has been this way for a long time, and it will continue. Whatever is difficult will be no more when we truly bring the truth of life in its divine expression into action.

238

Returning to Rosebud to dance, I regained connection with my uncle who asked for my help at the Hollow Horn Bear Sun Dance. I also reconnected with many of my immediate relations because I now had a two-week period every summer where I could go and be with the people. This reconnection with the people at Rosebud was a reaffirmation of all the things that I had been learning all my life. (I am still learning, and probably will learn more from my relations as I proceed along my life's journey.)

I had many friends who were not Lakota. A few Catholic priests, a few ministers, a few Mormon elders, who in my interaction with them would always get into a discussion of philosophy, worldview, cosmology. I also grew up with buddies who were like brothers of mine. They were not Lakota, but true brothers in that we experienced the hardships, the joys, and the growing pains of life at our time spent together at Rosebud. One of the things that always struck me in my interactions with the non-Lakota people was that they were my relations at the most profound spiritual level. Whether I agreed with what they believed in or not, I truly understood from all the teachings that I had that they, too, were my relatives.

I learned from my singing partners, friends, and relatives that when we begin to express our best sides in life, the worst sides of our life also confront us. The worst sides of our being confront us to challenge our basic goodness. In the teachings I have had about sitting in the center, when you have truly brought your being, your character, your personality, to that point of great adaptability to meet anything that happens, that great understanding you have puts you in a very high position of influence and also susceptibility.

239

My elders told me that in living in this world, and especially in my interactions with my non-Lakota relatives, I should always have reason and penetrating clarity of judgment. This helps, they said, to drive aside ulterior or hidden motives. We always talked about life. How it is. What it is. There was always a need expressed by the world to have judgment that understood dark, weak, or evil motives.

My discussions with my non-Lakota relatives allowed me to look back at my own people and see that we really valued the powerful influences of great personalities that knew how to uncover and help break up those little intrigues, mysteries, and failures of humanity. From my viewing both the Lakota and non-Lakota ways and behaviors, I could see clearly that all people have those who do not have light in them, but they could be uncovered, and they could be dealt with appropriately. This can be done through a great adaptability to life. I saw that we should not attempt to control life, but to actually move with it, to get in the flow with it. This improves life.

What I learned in my interaction with my relatives was the extreme of knowing how to adapt to most of the conditions that I encountered, but I learned also, again through the urgings of my grandmother and some of the older people I knew at Rosebud, the governmental agency, that character achievement only means that you know how to deal with all things as they transpire. You must have a great adaptability and a great understanding that knows how to stay behind the scenes, but at the same time have great outward influence by modeling and by accepting your own faults, mistakes, and blameworthy actions and then, muster the courage to overcome them.

240

My grandma, when she used to say, "Go humble yourself and be careful," meant that when you have great understanding, this great understanding produces changes in your life and in other people very gradually and somewhat behind the scenes. "To have great understanding," she would say, "you don't try to grasp and control what you try to understand, but by contemplating and by taking each step of your understanding to its fulfillment, you gain an understanding of the world through this process. That doesn't change the world overnight, but the changes made from these understandings and little actions last longer. They're more complete.

"If you want to have lasting influence and complete understanding of this world," she would say, "you have to go after something that's good for you and the world you live in. This kind of understanding and small acts are only achieved if the direction remains consistent. Some people, your own people, might think of this as weakness," she would say, "but it's to have a cause, giving yourself over to others, that you can help bring order to the world." In our case it was either the community, the tribe, or the *Tiospaye* (family). It was also from my grandmother that I learned that your mind works in a way that if you constantly feed it a certain quality and image of goodness, and you do this consistently, that goodness and that image all of a sudden realizes itself and becomes manifest.

Through my studies in Western thought, I began to understand this as the power of suggestion. Suggestion, if it is done ceaselessly, always achieves its purpose. Suggestion is powerful because time is its field of action. Time is its tool, its instrument. Learning from her how to stay with something to its

241

completion also taught me that as one becomes the center of ceremony, not only must there be calmness and stillness, but also the thought of goodness and love should penetrate the soul of the people by that consistency with which you strive for it. So, it takes work. Work in mind (not hard, manual labor kind of work) to have a lasting influence brought about by great clarity, by understanding, and by affirmation, command positive and successful results.

When this affirmation and command is accepted by people as that which to model their action in accordance with, goodness and love become all the more possible. If we try to intimidate people, if we take aggressive action toward people to make them be good, or clear, we only succeed in causing them fear. We push them away. At the Sun Dance each summer, we work with great passions and desires of individuals who come into the center to try to regain life, a new direction, a resolution. But there is always a dissension, a disharmony that has to be overcome because everyone comes as a warrior into the circle. In order to regain life, you have to put the warrior away to allow the spirit to express itself through your being again. When you do this, you become, literally, a living being again.

The paradox of the Sun Dance, to me, is that at the beginning, everyone has great hopes. Everyone who dances has the greatest desire for the end result of harmony, well-being, peace, and wisdom before we have done the work to actually get there. From what my grandmother taught me, as a leader, by taking each day as we begin a dance, we have to go through the process of uncovering those little intrigues, those little disharmonies, those little dissensions and disagreements as the process by which we get ever closer to harmony, and the end result of the spiritual expression of goodness and love.

And the paradox is that in order to start moving in that direction we always begin with the perseverance of that warrior to accomplish the goal in battle. It always has presented a wonderful paradox to me. If we are to get to the point of adaptability and to that point of gentleness as a spiritual expression, we have to deal with what the danger of that adaptability can bring. In achieving a very high state of clarity, understanding, adaptability, and gentleness, our understanding can bring us to a point of great indecision because our understanding sometimes fools us into thinking that our understanding will cause things to be better without the action being taken.

Indecision begins to create doubt. It begins to sap strength, and so forward movement toward this end goal of the virtue being expressed is sapped. People begin to lose their focus and strength in moving toward the goal they had in the first place. Doubts crop up. Dissension builds. No decision initially is made to stand firm with truth and goodness, so there is much drifting. Paradoxically, we, as leaders, often have to say to the people, "Be like the warrior to have the resolve and determination to move forward, but be willing to give that up at the point of adapting and experiencing harmony, peace, well-being, and wisdom!" It is amusing to use the very things that are to be overcome to try to get there. It is a true paradox to me.

The teaching, perhaps, is that in striving to achieve a great perfection of your being (which is a state of utter adaptability), discipline is much better than drifting, allowing yourself the license to do wrong things. This truth has always created in me

243

the understanding that when we drift away from this resolve, we have to do things paradoxically through action in the material to return to the way of peace and harmony.

What is meant by that? When we encourage people to move forward toward achieving perfection in character through their warrior ways, we encourage them to encounter obstructions, because the nature of aggressive strength attracts obstruction. By encouraging people to do this, we take that obstruction to the limit. It forces a return to a way suited to the situation, which in offering prayer and offering one's own possession, the body, back to spirit, helps one to let go of the will. The will that is full of desire, full of passion, is put away, so we return to the way in which we are free to move forward or to move backward. By taking things to the limit in this way, there is always a turn for the better because people see the extremes of what this brings. So, the initial goal of peace and harmony begins to prevail.

What one learns from this is that it is much wiser and more reasonable to obtain the good things by understanding and by the virtue of your actions rather than by trying to obtain these things by force. Every year, because we deal with warriors and warrior traditions to get to that point of having spirit find expression, we encounter much phenomena that in the Lakota worldview is common. These are experiences we grew up with. To the world at large these phenomena can be awesome, sometimes frightening, sometimes mysterious, sometimes bewildering, and sometimes confusing.

What that creates within individuals is that they begin to encounter what I would call their little hidden enemies, doubts, suspicions. Reactions and fear begin to create little doorways one opens in the psyche to let in external influences that go deep into the mind. They begin to cause disharmony and dissension. For those who have an aggressive nature, it causes greater aggression in the want to control one's own sense of power rather than influence. So, the conditions are set up where those intangible influences begin to affect people by suggestion. When you dance all day, you are expressing a willingness to let your being go back to creation. Yet, by the very process of dealing with those things you must put away, it becomes a process of suggestion. It becomes necessary to trace those things back to their most secret places, in order to determine their nature, so those things can be put away.

There are many within the circle of the Sun Dance who act as priests. Priests determine the nature of the influences to be dealt with. They speak to creation, to *Tunkasila,* of them as things to remove. Removing those influences becomes literally the job of the holy people, those who understand change and transformation, those who understand exactly how things work. By knowing the exactness with which this understanding shows these influences, they are dealt with in a very hidden, consistent effort that begins to remove them.

These influences become elusive when they are branded and brought into the open, and people act on them. But in their elusive qualities, their power of suggestion also begins to lose influence in their impact. In this process, those influences lose their power over people. The challenge then becomes one of helping people to understand that they have to return to a moral order that is built very consistently and slowly. It carries the danger that if you slow down, this order does not come any faster. But this consistency begins to change the whole mindset of the people. It is a very gradual process.

Sometimes misunderstanding can cut its own influences and be carried so far to the other extreme that the power of decision needed gets crippled. Much of the teaching in the transitional part of the Sun Dance is to help people thoroughly ponder what has to be done, what has to be decided upon, and to act on that decision quickly when it is understood. But the more people deliberate without taking any action, the more they become subject to fresh doubts, fresh thoughts of unworthiness, and the danger of humiliation because the loss of the power to act is complete.

When this loss occurs, a great transition is caused where a battle between decadent forces and the good is waged. Loss becomes greater in that what was to be dealt with in the beginning gets compromised. If the good prevails, and a just decision gets made to continue the dance appropriately, the effort becomes more to express harmony. The leaders become more responsible to show this, and the leaders occasionally fall from it because they, too, are dealing with the very things that are shown to be dealt with. But as one goes through the transition, one has to understand that we can make mistakes in moving to that goal of harmony and unity of the people. So the leaders, the holy people, and those who have understanding, the singers, take their positions responsibly and take their experience of many years of doing these things, and take energetic action toward that which has to be accomplished. With some humility, we always get to the end result of greatness.

As you stand in the center, what you begin to understand is that you have to offer your actions, in goodness and love, to *Tunkasila,* toward your relations who stand in the circle with you, and to those who are supporting on the sides of the dance. You must muster a willingness to do this every day, until you get to that end goal. When your efforts answer all three purposes of meeting your needs, meeting the needs of others, and meeting *Wakan Tanka's* needs, your hunt for that which is correct and appropriate is achieved. It comes at the point where you reunite the people to the celebration of song and of the dance. Unifying and harmonizing in a common effort to that high ideal which you set, you realize that your willingness to work toward it step-by-step, day by day, has been rewarded. You know that the reward comes from helping people to lay aside egotism, cupidity, to disperse the energy that gets blocked when we begin to have doubts and dissension. This dispersion begins to help regain the flow of energy and life and express it through that harmonious and harmonic movement of song and dance.

When all ego is laid aside and the individual becomes one with the group, mutual support of offering and sacrifice with individual acts begin to dissemble aggression and conflict. And if one maintains aggression and conflict throughout the dance, they create greater and greater isolation. So, the individual leaves the dance without having accomplished much.

My grandfathers, in my times with them either hunting or going after wild turnips or wood, always presented me with some lessons about being consistent and doing right things, so that mistakes could be removed by great action and understanding. When situations are encountered where something cannot be changed, my grandpas always used to say, "You have to take a whole new direction, a whole new road, to get away from those things. If small actions can reform the situation, it is good to do those things. When beginnings and united effort haven't been good, but you can take a new direction within it that brings change and improves the conditions, it's always good to take those steps. However, be committed to them so that you have a firm and appropriate and right attitude within your mind. The new direction you take will accomplish the purpose of uniting, and mistakes will disappear!"

With my Grandpa Robert Little Hawk, I went on a wagon trip to get wood. He was telling me to be cautious. He was saying, "There's rattlesnakes out here. There's animals. We're going to load this wagon, and it's going to become heavy. Loading wood onto the wagon takes work. You might get slivers. You could drop something and hurt yourself. I just want you to be careful. Let's try to do this right." And so I followed his lead.

We drove the wagon and the horses up onto a small butte overlooking a deep canyon on one side. Getting the wood on the ground and taking dead branches off the trees, we had the wagon half loaded in a short time. As the wagon became more full and heavier, Grandpa decided to drive it closer to the edge of the butte. Parking the wagon near the edge of the canyon side, we would walk down into the shallow draw of the canyon. We would pick the heavier pieces of wood and carry them up the side of the butte, up to the top of the butte, and throw them into the wagon.

On one occasion I came up in front of the horses out of the draw. At the same time, my grandpa came up behind the horses. He had a huge log. As he'd had difficulty carrying it up the side of the hill, he wanted to be rid of it. So, he got up to the wagon. He heaved the heavy log onto the wagon. It was a little heavier than other logs on the wagon, so it made a louder sound than usual as it landed on top of the other wood. The horses got frightened by the sound. I happened to be coming right in front of the wagon when I saw the horses take a running start at me, so I tried to jump out of the way. I had an armload of medium-sized pieces of wood that I had been hacking off the trees. I did not quite make it away from the full gallop of the horses; I fell and the first wheel of the wagon went over my leg. As I tried to move, the back end of the wagon went over both of my legs. I was laid face first on the ground looking away from my grand-father. I started to laugh. While I was laughing, my whole body was shaking. My grandpa came running to me. He had this sound of fear in his voice as he was asking me if I was all right. As he came to me, he very gently touched me from behind. He looked at my face. I saw a little speck of a tear in his eye. Meanwhile, I couldn't stop myself from laughing! When he saw that I was laughing, he started to laugh. We had a good long laugh.

After we finished laughing, he said, "Now that you're okay, now that I know that you're okay, I can laugh with you. You looked awfully foolish!" He started laughing again. "This is not your fault," he said, "but you should remember that you never go in front of horses, especially when there's others coming up behind them. Hooked to a wagon like this, they can frighten easily. I should have told you this!"

And we laughed. We laughed for quite a few minutes. We would stop, then start again. Once we finally stopped laughing for good, he asked me if I was really okay, if I was not hurt. I said, "No, but I'm surprised! I was laughing at myself because I threw that pile of wood back down the canyon. It took me awhile to get it up here!" And we started laughing again.

He called me *Takoja,* which means grandchild. "*Takoja,* it's good to learn how to deal with these horses. They are animals. They respond to their world as animals. They have an understanding within their own world, but they don't often understand us," he said, "and sometimes, we don't understand them, so we do something that frightens or startles them. You haven't been taught how to be careful . . . you did nothing wrong, but you could have been hurt. It's important," he raised his voice a little, "that you learn things about being careful. That you really, carefully consider how to stay safe and secure in any situation that you find yourself.

"If you want to know how to be safe and secure, think things through. Take care that what you are thinking is about right things. Do this over and over again, until you really understand that doing the right thing in a situation is what is needed and you have to act in that way all the time. When you have learned these things, these ways of knowing, this knowledge that you gain has to be acted on time after time so that it holds effect in your life." He would continue, "That kind of care always keeps you in good things, and if you can't make changes like this, things get pretty bad sometimes. That usually happens because sometimes, we refuse to listen to the world around us, from the elders, from our friends, or from the Spirit World. When we don't listen things truly, truly fall apart. Then we have to start things all over again to regain some care and caution about life. It's so important, *Takoja,* that you know this." And he pointed with his nose down the canyon, "Here, I'll help you get the wood you threw back down the canyon." So we walked back down the canyon and picked it all up. We put it in the wagon, and he said,

"We should go home now, this is enough excitement for this day." We went home with a good story.

What I learned about that, aside from the laughter, is that the impact of parents and grandparents, those who came before us, can be both good and bad. But we're given, as individuals, a will to begin to understand what is good and what is evil, and the gray area that exists between those two extremes. Our understanding is sufficient, always, to know what to choose. We can choose to remain in the dark about things. Or we can choose to take that which is given by our parents and grandparents, apply our own will to those capabilities and tendencies we are given by them to correct our own world. The things that can be corrected by us as individuals are those things that we do ourselves, where we corrupt and abuse our own freedoms. Those things that we do, we can absolutely correct because all it requires is work and decisions to make the effects of that work be evident in our daily living. Those things that happen to us we can always meet as individuals who should be pure and innocent, but those things that we corrupt, we are in positions to constantly correct them.

My grandfather was so determined that I knew this about human behavior that I felt I had learned that one very well. Again, using the power of suggestion, constantly convincing an affirmation to your mind about doing good and positive things will always have good results.

Christina and my Grandma Mary used to say that when we look backward into life and find only the bad things, we're going to get only the bad things in life. If your understanding allows you to look forward and know that good things can be,

251

because you choose to be good and to do good things, good things will follow. They used to warn me that if you always look to your past to conjure up that which has injured you, you succeed in finding these things in every dark corner of your mind. If you do this repeatedly, you'll lose your strength to fight those things, and you'll lose your ability to act in appropriate ways to balance your world. The more you get seduced into looking into your own darkness, the more you harm yourself.

They once told me that sometimes we bounce back and forth between looking to the past and finding all the injuries and dark things we did, and only succeed in holding ourselves in guilt. "The only thing that breaks the pattern," they both used to say, "is if you share your goodness, act in good and loving ways to your world, you bring great blessing to your people and to all people. If you share this without any boundary except that which is good, you move away from the injury of your past, and you gain the health and well-being of your future."

So, again, these were great lessons that I learned from my elders and from growing up with the Lakota people. In the Sun Dance, we go through all the struggles, the dissension, disharmony, working with people's passions, their weaknesses, and their strengths. It takes four days to get to that point of harmony. On the last day, not only is the thrill of having completed the dance swelling up and building, but also an actual healing has occurred. The people live again. What we started with as a goal at the beginning of the dance gets achieved by the end of the dance, and people celebrate again. Instead of dancing in prayer, they dance in celebration. They give to each other. They share. And it is so important to do those things in utter sincerity and honesty.

19

I Speak Sacredly;
Do Not Deceive Me!

Wicahpi Wankatuya!	High Star!
Le miye lo!	This is who I am!
Ognas,	Perhaps,
Mayagnaye ke lo!	You will deceive me!
He wakan ya,	Sacredly,
Iwaye lo!	I speak!
Ognas,	Perhaps,
Mayagnaye ke lo!	You will deceive me!
Canunpa wan,	A pipe,
Nica u pelo!	They are bringing to you!
Tanyan yuza yo!	Hold it well!
Ognas,	Perhaps,
Mayagnaye ke lo!	You will deceive me!
He wakan ya,	Sacredly,
Iwaye lo!	I speak!

Ognas,	Perhaps,
Mayagnaye ke lo!	You will deceive me!
Canunpa wan,	A pipe,
Unpin kte lo!	He will smoke it!
Tanyan unpa yo!	Smoke it well!
Ognas,	Perhaps,
Mayagnaye ke lo!	You will deceive me!
He wakan ya,	Sacredly,
Iwaye lo!	I speak!
Ognas,	Perhaps,
Mayagnaye ke lo!	You will deceive me!

254

The point of sincerity in all ceremony is that in reconnecting ourselves to the spirit, we are connecting with the spirit within, that which we are. The song that often closes my ceremonies is the song that a majority of those who do what I do use as the *Kinape Olowan* (Closing Song). In it, what becomes important is to name myself, because this is who I am. Also, in the song I must acknowledge that through my own self-deception, I can perceive the spirit being able to deceive me. But I learn the greater truth, that if I am to act and do things in a state of sincerity and integrity, I must demand and expect the same of the spirit. You must do the same—demand and expect sincerity and integrity of yourself and spirit.

Can the Spirit World deceive you? Our grandfathers and those who sat in the center before me say that everything happens in pairs. There is a light, and there is a dark. If we do not hold our relationship appropriately within and with all things, and consequently, do not hold an appropriate relationship with the spirit that is without and coexistent with the life we are living at the present, the dark side can enter. The dark side certainly will deceive you, seduce you. It will pull you into that which is seen almost as bright as goodness, but is very dark in nature. So, you say to the Spirit World that if you truly are expressing your divinity, your holiness, you are speaking sacredly and you are sacred. Yes, the Spirit World can deceive if it comes from the dark side.

In Lakota, when we offer a pipe to another individual, we are asking for a relationship that has commitment to get to an end result that is favorable to all. Consequently, when a person offers to me a pipe to do a ceremony or ritual, my choice at that moment is to accept it or to refuse it. I have the choice to accept relationship or to reject relationship.

When we offer a pipe to the Spirit World, we are asking for a reaffirmation of our relationship and a commitment that extends both ways, so we must hang onto the meaning of that pipe in a very good way. Maybe by self-deception, I can allow the Spirit World to speak to me in deception. Perhaps I might deceive myself and speak deceptively to the Spirit. On the other hand, if I smoke this pipe, believe, act, and walk within the virtues that it stands for, the smoking of the pipe is to allow the prayer to go into the realm of the invisible. The prayer will find consecration and take firm root in the appropriate order of all things. So smoking the pipe is akin to saying, "Pray well." Yes, the Spirit World can deceive me, but I speak sacredly.

The education I have had from the old people in the world around me, including all my friends, and the schooling I have had in the Western tradition, have given nourishment to this rational mind of mine. Much of those teachings have found

255

a great challenge as well as difficulty in life for me. But if I were to look back at my whole life as a process, not a logical step-by-step process, but as a matter of growth and development, what could I say that I have found in this writing that is to be about healing?

Healing is a matter of balancing forces so that life is renewed at every turn of our action and reaction. This truth has led me to the belief that the foundation of humanity is the same in everyone, not only in Lakota people, but in all people. The process I learned from the sacred ways, the Spirit World, and just in living day to day, is that there is a way to be in balance. There is a way to live your life as a meaningful expression of the divine. That is what is real, and the rest is an illusion. We are always shaping the illusion according to our desires and our passions. I sit here now. I look back at this as a process. What have I learned?

Anytime we begin a journey, an endeavor, a spiritual path, or enter a spiritual opening, we have to sit down and deal with our passions and our desires. We must learn how to start behaving appropriately to begin to harmonize with the relationships within self and within the organic world. By harmonizing efforts, through appropriate behavior with others, the purpose of harmony starts to be achieved. This purpose is to get to an end result of uniting forces so great things can be accomplished. But in that process a change must occur in the attitude of mind to balance the extremes of life. What my grandmother called "humbling yourself." Humbling oneself allows one to learn to honor truth. In that truth, it becomes necessary to learn how to love.

If I applied this process to myself, what would I say? I learn how to support my weaknesses with strength and to tone down my strengths so that they do not overstep boundaries. I begin to examine myself in terms of the effects I have on the world, so that I can know myself. If anything, I should know myself better than I know other people and other things in my life.

Only in this way will I find that light within myself that will allow me to honor and return to an expression of the divine, which is an intrinsic part of my own nature and in the nature of all things. If I find this light, I can return to goodness, goodness being the foundation of all that grows and develops appropriately.

My grandfathers, in their many teachings, say that we only have true power from the spiritual side. It is expressed in two ways. The first is, we are given the power to correct fault, the means to do good. The other is the power to love, which is to attract all that is appropriate and meant for you into your life. This unity with that which is meant for you can leave great things behind on the path that you walk.

257

In order to do those great things that can be done in life, we have to look at the very things that we are given by our parents. The things that I develop as an individual within my own capabilities and understanding is only half of my life. The other half is given a direction by what my parents have given to me. If I act within that understanding, there will be a consistency in how I achieve my purposes and goals in life. I can only do that if I put the very things that I started with away, to give my will back to creation, to Grandfather and to Grandmother. I must learn to put my anger aside so that I can bring passion to stillness. I must put a restraint on my instincts, curb them as best as I can, so that I keep nourishing and feeding the higher parts of my soul. I must also learn to take this in service to the world. Not to try to manipulate it, not to try to bind it or attach it to me or my desires and passion, but to give all honor to the spirit that alone has power to help the world. If I learn to give service in this way, I learn to look at the world around me. I learn to imitate the good things in it, and change the bad I see in the world in myself so that I can serve it better. When I am tested by life, I learn that these are just parts of life itself, so instead of having spite for it and blaming the world for it, I accept it. I take my will and stake my life on it because I know I will get through the test. Doing this will put me back into proper relationship with the world where I can influence it in such ways that people will work together. And I can encourage others to do better work than they show, that they can strive for the kind of perfection that will endure.

258

Above all, if I learn truly to be gentle with myself, then I can love myself as the expression of the divine. Then I can share this love with the rest of the world and handle all things that occur within me and occur without me. If I do this completely with integrity, I will not have to put myself in front of the people, and try to lead them. I can influence them from behind the scenes so they can go do great things. "Remove the intrigues, manipulations, and obstacles of life" my people have told me. I believe them. If we constantly do this in small ways, gently, with great understanding, the world will find peace, harmony, justice, and wisdom. That is what I see as the process of becoming a whole person. When you are a whole person, you do not go seek healing from others. If you are not a whole person at this time, and you need that help, the sacred people, the Spirit World, and the spirit within yourself is present and omnipresent at all times to call upon for this help.

So, yes! Healing is a balancing of the forces that can renew your life every single moment. As a person who sits at the center of many ceremonies, I encourage the true work that is healing. That is what I hope to influence others with throughout my life.

We are at the end of our ceremony. You, the reader, have entered a relationship, a prayer, an affirmation as well as the supplication of good in love. In this prayer, if you have prayed for yourself and for others, you'll find that this ceremony was a door opening for you to love yourself. You cannot really love others unless you love yourself. By opening this door, you learn to do good for yourself, for others, and for the Spirit World, so the purposes of the Great Spirit can be fulfilled.

At the end of our ceremony, we usually feed each other. If you happen to be the one asking for this ceremony, you would have a giveaway; you would share things with those who were in the ceremony with you. Sitting at the center of ceremony, I do not demand these things as rules of behavior. I suggest to you, however, that when you lay this book down, you go and feed someone. Give someone some food, share some drink, but nourish someone spiritually also. Share your goodness, your love. As a giveaway, go give someone something that they can use to benefit their lives, or simply do an act of kindness, just because it comes from your heart to do this. You will see the practical side of what this ritual and ceremony has helped you with. So I suggest that you do this.

A further suggestion I have is that instead of becoming dependent on ritual and ceremony to understand goodness and love, find every moment that you can to act in goodness. Act in loving ways, simply because it is there to be done. And you will

259

put yourself on the same path that I have been on to learn the things I have learned. You can know and do the same things I have done because they are there to be done.

Talking with the Spirits is a role that those of us who are given this responsibility take seriously. Because this responsibility requires sincerity, I say without shame or compunction that this is what I do sitting in the center of ceremony. Outside of the center, I live my life as simply and easily as I can. I forgive myself for the mistakes I make, for I am human. I encourage myself when I do good things because it is only appropriate to do good things. I strive to love all, not to embattle myself with evil, but to work energetically in the progress of the good so that good will prevail.

The Way of the Pipe is meant to bring peace, harmony, well-being, and wisdom to our people. I have been taught to share what this is with the world so that *Tunkasila, Wakan Tanka,* find expression in the same ways in the world.

This is the end of our ceremony. I encourage you to go live. Go live well! And I encourage you, when you need help, ask for it. When you can give help, give it with goodness and love.

We are done. *Mitakuwe Oyas'in.*

RESOURCES

Black Bear, Ben, Sr., and R. D. Theisz. *Songs & Dances of the Lakota.* Rosebud, S.D.: Sinte Gleska College, 1976.

Brown, Joseph E., ed. *The Sacred Pipe: Black Elk's Account of the Seven Rites of the Oglala Sioux.* Norman, Okla.: University of Oklahoma Press, 1989.

Bucko, Raymond A. *The Lakota Ritual of the Sweat Lodge: History and Contemporary Practice.* Lincoln, Nebr.: University of Nebraska Press, 1998.

Buechel, Eugene. *A Grammar of Lakota: The Language of the Teton Sioux Indians.* Rosebud, S.D.: Rosebud Educational Society, 1939.

Buechel, Eugene, and Paul Manhart, eds. *The Lakota-English Dictionary.* Pine Ridge, S.D.: Holy Rosary Mission, 1970.

DeMallie, R. J., ed. *The Sixth Grandfather: Black Elk's Teachings Given to John G. Neihardt.* Lincoln, Nebr.: University of Nebraska Press, 1984.

Densmore, Frances. *Teton Sioux Music and Culture.* Lincoln, Nebr.: University of Nebraska Press, 1992.

Hyde, George E. *Spotted Tail's Folk: A History of the Brulé Sioux.* Norman, Okla.: University of Oklahoma Press, 1961.

Neihardt, John G. *Black Elk Speaks.* N.Y.: Pocket Books, Simon & Schuster, Inc., 1959.

Powers, William K. *Oglala Religion*. Lincoln, Nebr.: University of Nebraska Press, 1977.

————. *Sacred Language: The Nature of Supernatural Discourse in Lakota*. Norman, Okla.: University of Oklahoma Press, 1986.

————. *Yuwipi: Vision and Experience in Oglala Ritual*. Lincoln, Nebr.: University of Nebraska Press, 1982.

Theisz, R. D. "Acclamations and Accolades: Honor Songs in Lakota Society." *Kansas Quarterly* 13, no. 2 (Spring 1981): 27–43.

————. "The Bad Speakers and the Long Braids. The Depiction of Foreign Enemies in Lakota Song Texts." In *Indians and Europe*, edited by Christian Feest. Aachen, West Germany: Rader Verlag, 1987.

————. "A Case of Neglecting the Conspicuous: Teaching American Indian Music." *Wassaja* 5 (September 1977).

————. "The Critical Collaboration: Introductions as a Gateway to the Study of Native American Bi-Autobiography." *American Indian Culture and Research Journal* 5, no. 1 (1981): 65–80.

————. "Identity Through Song: The Increasingly Dominant Role of Music and Dance in Lakota Society." Presented at the Center for Great Plains Studies Symposium, University of Nebraska/Lincoln, March, 1986.

————. "The Interest in the American Indian: Voyeurism or a Case of Sweetness and Light." Black Hills State College Faculty Interdisciplinary Seminar, April, 1978.

————. *Lakota Art Is an American Art: Readings in Contemporary and Traditional Sioux Art* (4 vols.). Spearfish, S.D.: Black Hills State College, 1980.

————. "The Multifaceted Double Woman: Legend, Song, Dream and Meaning." *The European Review of Native American Studies* 2, no. 2 (1988): 9–15.

————. "Powerful Feelings Recollected in Tranquility: Literary Criticism and Lakota Social Song Poetry." *Great Plains Quarterly* 20, no. 3 (2000): 197–210.

————. "Red Leaf Singers, Classic and Live" (Review) *Lakota Times*, September 24, 1986, 3.

————. *Sending Their Voices: Essays on Lakota Musicology*. Kendall Park, N.J.: Lakota Books, 1996.

————. "Singing as Identity Assertion in Lakota Life." Presented at Dakota State College, Madison, History Conference, 1985.

————. "Social Control and Identity in American Indian Humor" *Studies in Contemporary Satire* 16 (1989).

———. "Song Texts and Their Performers: The Centerpiece of Lakota Identity Formation." *Great Plains Quarterly* 7, no. 2 (Spring 1987): 116–124.

———. "Teaching Native American Bi/Autobiography." Presented at the Modern Language Association Convention, Denver, 1978.

Theisz, R. D., ed. *Buckskin Tokens: Contemporary Lakota Oral Narratives.* Aberdeen, S.D.: North Plains Press, 1975.

Walker, James R. *Lakota Belief and Ritual.* Edited by R. J. DeMallie and E. Jahner. Lincoln, Nebr.: University of Nebraska Press, 1980.

Young Bear, Severt, and R. D. Theisz. *Standing in the Light. A Lakota Way of Seeing.* Lincoln, Nebr.: University of Nebraska Press, 1994.

Note from the author:
Song renditions and texts for *Native American Healing* are available from High Star Productions, Inc., P.O. Box 3069, Taos, NM 87571; (505) 758-8916.

ABOUT THE AUTHOR

Howard P. Bad Hand is a Sicangu Lakota from Rosebud, South Dakota, and was educated at The Lenox School, Dartmouth College, Harvard University, and Sinte Gleska College.

Raised in a family of singers, he has become a well-known singer and composer of songs in the Lakota tradition as well as the lead singer of Red Leaf Takoja and Heart Beat singing groups. He gives workshops and seminars worldwide on Native American singing and has translated books and articles on the Lakota language into English.

Bad Hand currently works as an intuitive consultant, teaching and coaching individuals on the path of spiritual development and on the use of the *I-Ching* as a manual for self-development. He also owns High Star Productions, Inc., which produces cassettes and videos of Native American music and dance performances. He resides with his family in Taos, New Mexico.